GRACE IN MOVEMENT

Grace in movement

THE TRAINING OF YOUR ENERGY CHANNELS FOR BETTER HEALTH AND PERFORMANCE

Dr Jerzy Dyczynski MD

dyczynskitelehealth.co

For my wonderful wife Angela and our daughter Fatima Dyczynski,
an Aerospace Engineer

Contents

1

Introduction

1. Introduction

When you read this text, you have initiated a transformation from a three-dimensional oriented person to a spiritual being interconnected with grace and linked to the fabric of the Universe. It is a pathway to becoming a more energetically motivated and healthier person.

The study of your own body and its energy channels is a key to it. Every energy channels is connected to your brain, heart, and spinal cord. The solar plexus in the belly around your gut, and the pelvic plexus below the tummy button link heart, brain and spine with the most of energy channels, according to 21st-century medical research.

The major sensory and motor nerves provide the pathways for energy channels. The information between nerve cells and neurons is transmitted wirelessly by means of the electromagnetic waves through structures on their surface, similar to antennas. The antennas are meeting points of your wireless commands from the mind to the cells. Then, the nerve roots transmit the impulses to the muscles via electrical currents. This wireless communication is ongoing and intensifies when you voluntarily accelerate your breathing or relax your muscles.

The communication and the vital energy flow freely alongside your body and concentrate at the entry points to the energy channels They are the gateway points that establish the interface between the outside and inside of your body. The entry points have exceptional sensors (receptors) and a rich blood vessel network connecting them directly to the heart and brain. They regulate the energy exchange in your body and guard its integrity.

Your body is a self-organizing system and can tune up and tune down the flow of vital energy, its intake and distribution. It creates a bidirectional flow of bio-impulses, one stream of information from outside to the inside and another flow to your environment.

2

The essentials for energy channel training

Your body has a robust structure in the three-dimensional world, but its appearance and functionality can anytime change. It is a good functioning self-organizing system. The heart and brain are associated with the energy channels and wireless with your mind. Your intelligent heart and smart brain are the engines for your inspired energy channel training. You will train also your awareness of your energy channels location and how they run alongside your muscles.

Your energy channel training will focus on physical training of your muscles. The awareness training of your abdominal breathing, the movements of the diaphragm, will support the continuous contact with the spinal cord, the solar and pelvic plexus. You will experience during your training that your body has a unique orbit similar to the orbit of our planet Earth.

The training of your energy channels will improve the regulation at the interface between the outside and inside of your body. Energy channel training will create more resilience and a new smooth, graceful pattern for your movements. Your trained body will be then more flexible, radiant, and attractive, and a striking drawing power will appear in your outer expression. This distinct new appeal of you becomes noticeable because your mind and spirit can express themselves better through your trained body. The energy channel training will increase your intellectual and physical well-being.

Think about it: your body is wonderful. The laws of gravity act on your body at all times. Despite of gravity, it can be highly flexible and sometimes seems to be very hard, like iron.

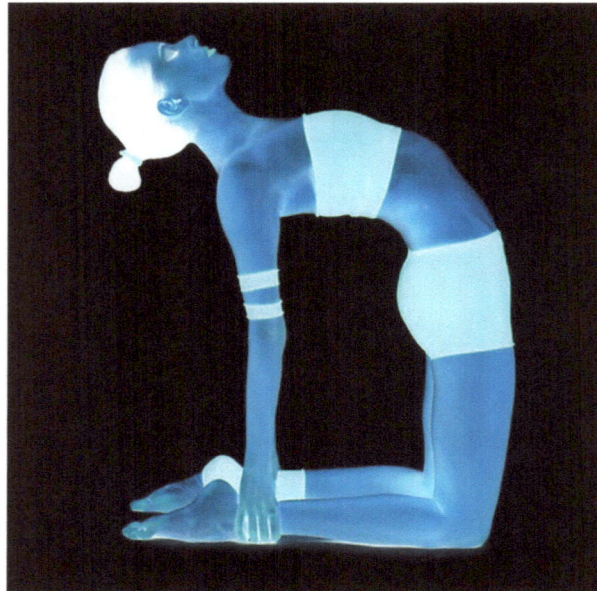

Picture 1. Ustrasana by Nina Mel, Yoga Teacher
By Kennguru - Own work, CC BY 3.0,
https://commons.wikimedia.org/w/
index.php?curid=25670620

Your mind and spirit can rest inside your body during your training, as shown by the yoga practitioner Nina Melat in the photograph above or your mind and spirit can be fully active and deployed to the field outside your body as it is illustrated in the picture below by the determined action of Steven Ho performing the martial arts.

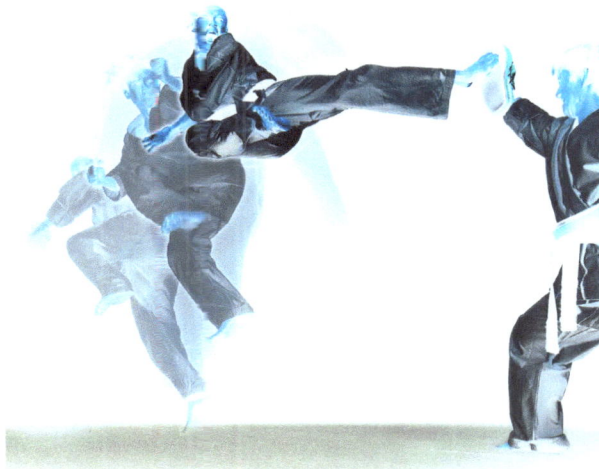

**Picture 2 Steven Ho executing a Jump Spin Hook Kick.
Steven Ho: Jump Spin Hook Kick. Martial Artist Steven
Ho kicks a focus mitt. Steven Ho, martial artist and
action choreographer.**
Wikipedia user Nt2bd, CC BY-SA 3.0,
https://commons.wikimedia.org/w/index.php?curid=8073618

The energy channel training will also prepare you for negative scenarios when the entry points become overloaded or overpowered with informational impulses, toxic or traumatic impact. These adverse effects will cause a slowing down of the energy flow. In this situation, the entry points will transmit less of vital energy, or they will block it as a protective and preventative measure.

At the same time body's self-organizing system will decrease the metabolism in this region of your body. It will result in stagnation symptoms like swelling and pain. The constricted blood vessels in the concerned area will cause insufficient oxygenation of the tissues and inadequate water exchange. Stagnated water in the cells accumulates the wastes of the changed metabolism and lactic acid, causing pain and stiffness. The disturbed flow of vital energy can temporarily restrict your body's functionality.

The limitation in movements will inform you that you need to rest, and visible signs of inflammation can appear. However, this negative impact can be reversed by stimulating the gateway points and restoring the flow of vital energy. Specific energetic training of your channels, an intervention with acupuncture, gentle massage, or local application of essential oils can support the opening of the constricted blood vessels.

The discovery of orbital breathing, a technique where you sense and visualize your breath moving in a circular path, is a life-changing experience.

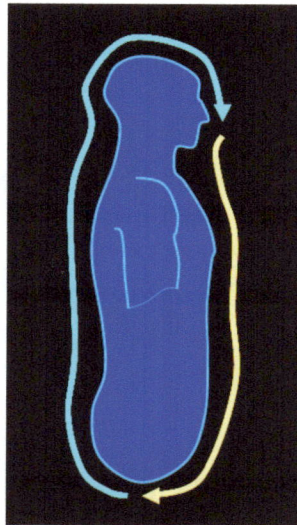

Picture 3 Simplified version of the micro-cosmic orbit.
By Bostjan46 - Own work, CC0.https://commons.wikimedi a.org/w/ index.php?curid=18986673

This practice, akin to your breath rotating alongside your own bodily orbit, will elevate your vital energy to a higher level. Sometimes, during orbital breathing, you will experience an energy shower, a burst of energy all over your body, starting from your head and shoulders and descending to your toes.

Increasing awareness or self-awareness of the interior of your body helps you realize the importance of your heart and brain and their connection to the energy channel pathways.

With your training progress, you will feel the vitality streams in your energized body. It can eventually merge into an integrative quantum experience, a new quality in the feeling of your body. When you reach it once, you will know you can repeat this experience. This new perception of your body will be a joyful part of your orbital breathing activity and energy channel training. Remember, where attention goes, the energy flows.

Your orbital breathing serves as a powerful reminder of your divine connection to the electromagnetic field of the fabric of the Universe. The moment you achieve integration with it, it becomes an inspiration, showing you that you can initiate this profound experience again and again. It will fill your life with more joy.

Your consistent energy channels training will give you further insights about your invisible components, the mind and spirit, and how are intensely entangled with your body as well as muscles. When your mind and spirit are united, perfectly cooperating with your internal organs and muscles, it will create grace in your body. When your mind, spirit, and body work in harmony, it creates a graceful smoothness and elegance in your movements. Remember, the WHOLE is greater than the sum of its parts.

Translating the grace of the universe to a personal level is a spiritual quest. Achieving unity between the body, heart, mind, spirit and soul is a profound mystery.

Your defining moment is the empowering decision to embark on your energy channel training. This choice, regardless of your current health or activity level, holds the potential for significant progress. Whether you are already balanced and healthy or have some physical weak points, the journey you are about to undertake will undoubtedly elevate your strength and your well-being.

3

The environment for your training

You must engage with your body and the environment, no matter whether you are agile or mobile. The gravitational world is constantly weighing on you. Your visible physical shape, known as the human body, exists in the 3D world and can be seen, photographed, and looked at in the mirror. Everybody on this planet needs to improve spine function, as everyone has the potential to advance the heart and brain functionality. It is a gravitational challenge.

Both the heart and spine have to produce the thrust to overcome gravity. Well, overcoming the resistance and reaching the antigravity fitness will be integral to your training. Choose wisely the environment for your training. Natural energy waves are best known to your body, and nature knows them perfectly, too. The vicinity of a water-like blue ocean, river, or lake is an essential factor in your choice. Blue color signals high energy.

Outdoor training should be your preference because of its natural composition and analog character. The blue colors of the sky and blue waters represent the natural high energy sources, and you need to collaborate with them. Analog means something similar to something else. The human body and all of nature are functioning almost identically. What they have in common are the energy waves. Natural waves of water, the wirbelwind of air, and the blowing wind around your ears, the singing of birds, or the swishing sound of rustling leaves will be in tune with your heart, creating pulsating waves of blood. Natural analog sounds are pleasant and will be in accord with your rhythmical breathing initiating waves of movements in your body. Your oscillating blood pressure and the wave-like pattern of movements of your muscles will cooperate with the wind and water's waves.

I hope you like the blue sky as I do. You love the turquoise water in the ocean, as all do. But wait a moment; the water is not blue but a transparent liquid. Neither is the space above us blue; it is black. What makes the blue color in water and air? It is the high energy of light travelling at a speed higher than light measured in dark space. When light hits water or air, it creates a particular blue high-frequency radiation that makes the ocean's water turquoise and the air above all of us blue. This Nobel Prize rewarded the discovery of high-energy blue Cherenkov radiation in 1953.

By the way, the image of our planet Earth is a true blue. Look at this spectacular "blue marble" image below. This is the most detailed true-color image of the entire Earth to date. Using a collection of satellite-based observations, scientists and visualizers stitched together months of observations of the land surface, oceans, sea ice, and clouds into a seamless, true-color mosaic of every square kilometer of our planet. https://visibleearth.nasa.gov/view.php?id=57723, Public Domain, Wikipedia.

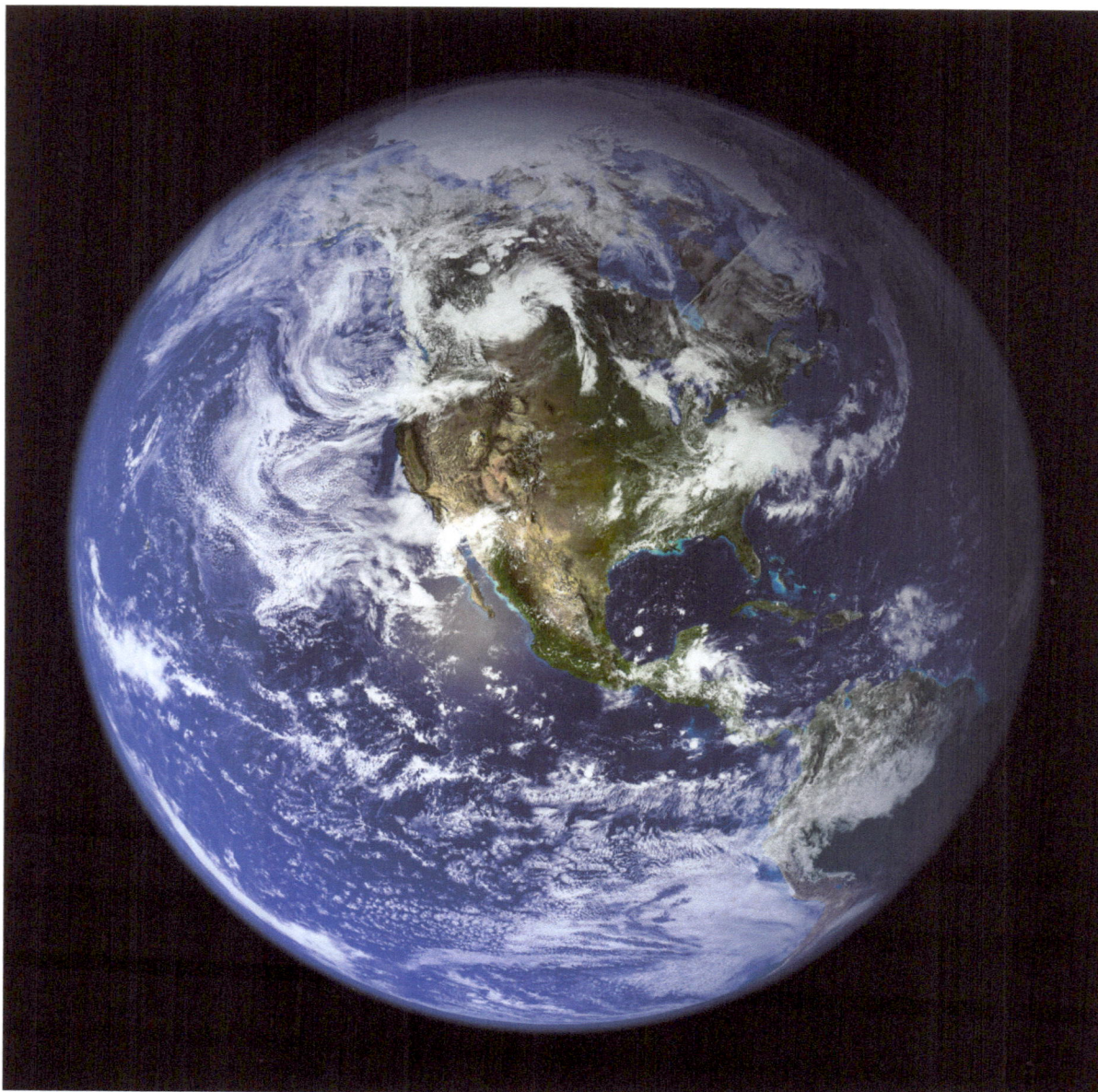

Picture 4. Blue, marble image of Earth from space. Credit: NASA.

4

Your personal grace

Physical training is good, but training for godliness is much better, promising benefits in this life and in the life to come. Timothy 4:8

The laws of physics, such as gravity, apply to the 3D world. You can move left or right, forward or backward, and up or down. Everything around you exists in three dimensions: height, length, and width. However, the laws of quantum physics and the Universe's electromagnetic field also influence the existence of your spiritual and invisible aspects

Albert Einstein said," The field is the only reality." Your invisible Wi-Fi connection to Einstein's electromagnetic field is a natural link. We all live in and are immersed in it. You interact with this field because your body generates electricity that flows through you and a magnetic field that surrounds you.

The recent adverse environmental impact on your health and well-being, the poor quality of air, and the micro plastic in Earth's waters prove that we all are interconnected in this 3D world. Yet, your soul and your spirit connect you with all human beings on this planet. Quantum entanglement provides a scientific demonstration that everything in the Universe is linked.

11

Recognition of this interconnectedness will lead you to care more about our Earth and the people. It will create a greater sense of empathy, compassion, and responsibility for their well-being.

As you journey through life, you will encounter the spiritual and bodily effects of your lifestyle, your decisions, and the outcomes of your actions in the world. Every energy you release into the universe, or share within Einstein's field will come back and support you, or it will backfire negatively and hit you like a boomerang. This is broadly known as the law of karma or the law of the spiritual consequences. It will significantly shape your health and your spiritual and intellectual well-being.

Maintaining grace in your movements within the field is a profound challenge and a spiritual quest that transcends the three-dimensional world. Remember, your energy channels are the bridge between the tangible parts of your body and your invisible mind and spirit.

There are several virtues in the beautiful qualities of your spirit, and you have all of them at your disposal from birth. Grace is one of them. Therefore, grace in movement is a contributing factor to your good self-esteem. It creates an uplifting feeling and can be a source of compliments in your social environment. When you move gracefully, it creates a feeling of joy in you.

Walking through the field produces friction in 3D, so how you move is of great importance. You can minimize the counteracting resistance by realizing you have your bodily energy channels connected to your muscles and can voluntarily relax them at any time. Full awareness of this will reduce the resistance and lead you to a better integration into the field and your environment. It will result in a good feeling for your body and a noticeable improvement in your bodily grace.

Grace in movement is not just about physicality, but also about the harmonious flow of life force in the energy channels of your body. Your unoccupied mind, free from double world's standards and the positive state of your spirit are powerful contributors to this flow. This attitude, which we can liken to a "silver line ", is something you can cultivate and strengthen during your energy channels training. It holds the potential to transform your movement and your life.

If you are searching for a model for your bodily grace, you can discover ballet and its energy field. A ballet dancer is a solid manifestation of it. Perfection in movement is often expressed in professional ballet dancing. Ballet movements are so beautiful that they can capture almost everybody's attention. Watching ballet dancers you feel a sense of awe. Their grace is not just a result of their training, but a reflection of their spiritual and physical discipline.

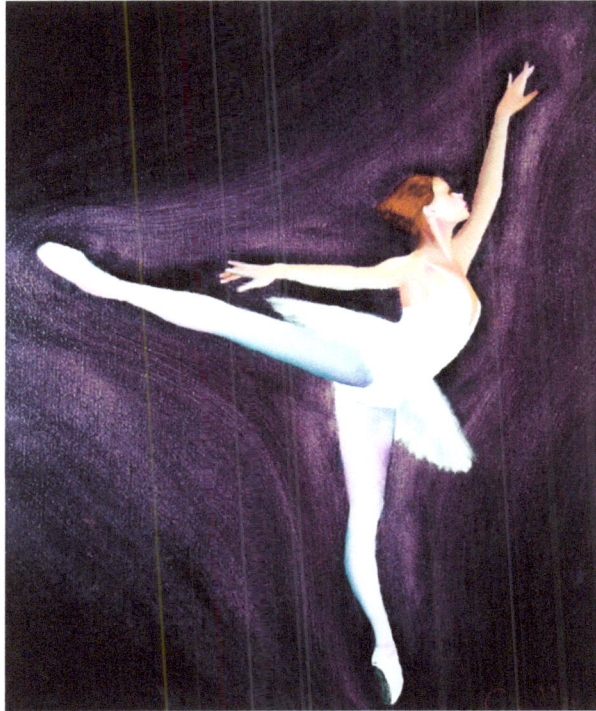

5 Ballerina oil painting by Flasher.
Wikipedia, CC BY-SA 3.0 , via Wikimedia Commons

The ballet dancer may awaken your desire to walk or move with similar perfection. What you admire is her well-trained body, unprecedented flexibility, and focused movements. You know that she is a professional dancer. You assume that she has trained for a long time. You anticipate her unique attitude of perseverance and physical stamina. She can be an excellent example of grace in movements. Her spiritual qualities, her focus and discipline, match her body's appearance in the 3D world of gravity. It's a reminder that graceful movements are not just about physicality, but also about the attitude of your mind and your spirit.

So, can you cultivate a similar quality of grace in movements? Absolutely, and energy channel training is the key. It's not an unattainable dream, but a goal within your reach. It may require some inspired actions on your part, but the potential is there for you to unlock.

5

Your bodily grace is the function of your heart and spirit

"Guard your heart above all else for it is source of life " Proverbs 4:23

The heart, the body's central organ, has been revered for its spiritual healing powers throughout history. This belief has also stood the test of time, persisting as a cornerstone of traditional medicines across cultures and generations. Traditional medical approaches, with their profound understanding of healing, recognize the intangible spirit residing within the human heart.

The World Health Organization (WHO) recognizes the significance of traditional medicine's long history. The practices, experiences, and beliefs that have been used in healing and maintaining health for thousands of years are a rich heritage that we continue to cherish in indigenous and modern cultures.

Practices used for healing and related to the heart in traditional medicines include:
•traditional European medicine,
•traditional Chinese medicine.
•alternative Ayurveda medicine
•traditional African medicine

•Korean and Person-Arabic medicine

The consideration of the human heart as a central organ to the body's functionality and its spiritual dimensions is a solid part of European traditional medicine, traditional Chinese medicine, and Indian Ayurveda medicine.

In Europe there is a very long history of traditional medicine that has a respectable historical and scientific dignity. In the 4th century before Christ, the renowned Greek philosopher Aristotle made a profound discovery about the human body. He identified the heart as the most essential organ, the first to form, based on his meticulous observations. Aristotle believed that the heart is the seat of intelligence, motion, and sensation. He described it as a chambered organ and the centre of vitality in the body, with other organs like the brain and lungs serving to cool it.

In traditional Chinese medicine, the heart is believed to be the most important organ for human health. Within the heart resides a spirit, which is the source of conscience. The heart also helps us maintain calmness, wellness, and general health while guiding us to distinguish between right and wrong. The heart is responsible for all creative activities and helps humans connect with the spiritual realm. It also influences our sleep pattern.

The Ayurveda alternative medicine system has its historical roots in the Indian subcontinent. It recognizes that the human heart consists of "two hearts". The physical heart pumps the blood and is in charge of entire circulation.

The other heart is an intangible one and it is emotional heart that experience joy, sadness and everything in-between. https://en.wikipedia.org/wiki/Traditional_medicine.

https://www.banyanbotanicals.com/info/ayurvedic-living/living-ayurveda/health-guides/vibrant-heart/ https://academic.oup.com/eurheartj/article/38/5/313/2990022

Also, Unani traditional medicine recognizes the heart as a chief organ of the human body.

https://www.ncbi.nlm.nih.gov/pmc/articles/PMC8217184/

Recent breakthroughs in cardiology, quantum physics, and medical physics have affirmed the heart's pivotal role in the human body, encompassing its connection to spirituality and memory.

Memory is one of the most sophisticated functions of humans, contributing significantly to one's personality. In a study published in 2000 the authors brought evidence of an existing link between the heart and human memory. It revealed that parts of a donor's personality and awareness go with a heart transplant to the recipient. This ground-breaking research transformed our understanding of the heart and its intelligence. Recipients of transplanted hearts were able to recall the specific life circumstances of the donors despite never having had any contact with them. This study represented a significant advancement in acknowledging the heart as an organ capable of inheriting memories.

These findings not only validate traditional spiritual beliefs but also establish a profound connection between ancient wisdom and modern cardiology, reassuring us of the compatibility of these two seemingly disparate medical approaches. This alignment of the traditional with modern medicine further strengthens the credibility of the spiritual beliefs in natural healing, offering a sense of unity in medicine.

6

The universal and common grace

The Bible is a bestseller and can serve as a focal point to understand the universal grace. Through abundant blessings, universal, common grace describes God's kindness to all people, believers and non-believers. Grace is a virtue from God and from the Universe, making you special and unique. It sets you apart from others. Grace is a way of life intertwined with health and integrity. It requires an active effort to maintain it, as it is important for you and me, not only for us, but also for the greater good.

Pope John Paul II, a significant figure in the Catholic Church during the 20th century, was not only a leader but also an avid athlete and sports fan. He became a patron saint of Catholic sports due to his profound love for sports. He urged athletes to strive for their full potential through exercise and training and to use sports to promote peace on Earth. In 1987, John Paul II described the universal grace in the encyclical "Redemptoris Mater" - Mother of the Redeemer.https://www.vatican.va/content/john-paul-ii/en/encyclicals/documents/hf_jp-ii_enc_25031987_redemptoris-mater.html

7

Heart's energy channel. Your intelligent heart and its spirit

"Because you are sons and daughters, God sent the Spirit of his Son into our hearts, crying, "Abba, Father!" Galatians 4:6

Your heart is at the core of your bodily perfections. The heart channel is the most important energy channel in your body. It is the principal organ contributing to your health, mobility and vitality. It needs a lot of oxygen to perform its multiple functions. Your heart energy channel primarily supports your brain, your internal organs, and your muscular movements. The heart energy channel guides your hands. Whatever your intention is born in your heart, your hands will perform it. Your heart interconnects all energy channels of your body.

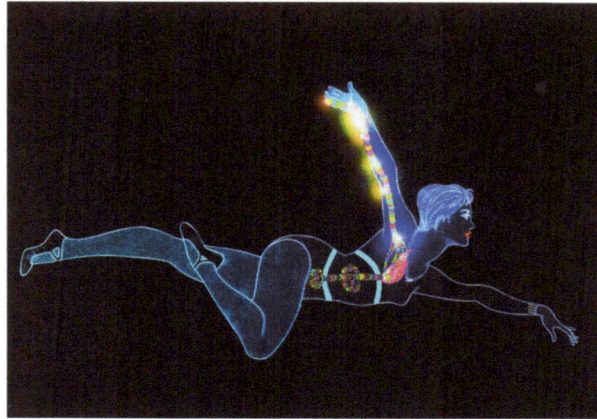

Picture 6. The heart energy channel. The internal branches connecting the heart channel to the eyes and solar as well as pelvis plexus are displayed. The gateway points are like nodes, marked with light. They are entrances for vital energy and information.
Own work.

Your heart is a profoundly spiritual organ and a highly contested place in your body. This fact has a rich representation in human history and culture. The metaphysical heart is, was, and will be the central organ of spirituality and healing in human beings, as it is in you. The intangible aspects of your being connected to the heart, including your emotions, thoughts, and intentions, are reflected in your intellectual activity, rest, and sleep, particularly in the pattern of your posture and movements.

Take solace in your heart. It is a tireless, dedicated, and empathetic organ. Your heart is a realm where love, trust, justice, wisdom, and grace converge. Your heart knows what is right. It distinguishes between the healthy and the unhealthy tendencies in your body and your environment.

Your heart actively engages with the fabric of the Universe. It allows you to experience more frequently a sense of all-inclusiveness, sometimes even a state of bliss. It happens when the heart governs all well functioning energy channels and integrates them into one perfect all-sensing system of your body. Many athletes, sports instructors, and renowned yogis who practice specialized physical training and meditation have also encountered this extraordinary state of unity. It is a unique blend of emotions: euphoria, calmness, contentment, serenity, and joy, acting in unison and simultaneously.

This potent state can be also identified by everyone who once has fallen in love. Everybody has had experienced such a time of universal unity of the body, soul, mind, heart, and spirit. It made an imprint in your memory as a transformative moment, a catalyst that elevated you to your infinite potential and inspired you to push your boundaries.

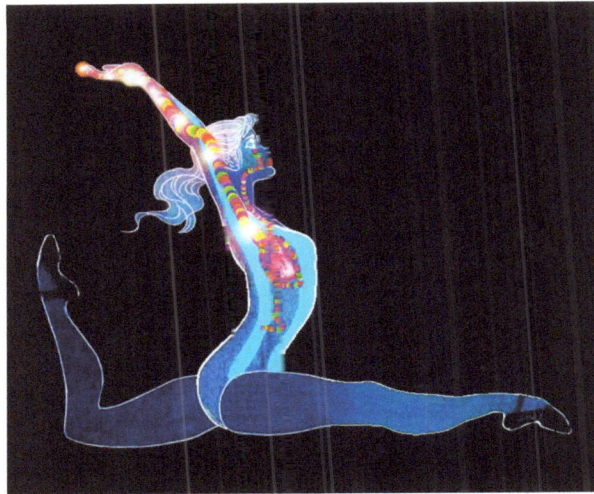

Picture 7. The heart energy channel starts at the heart and ends at the small finger. It has nine entry points, with the first one emerging from the armpit
Own work.

Your heart is always in motion; it never rests. During physical training, your heart tirelessly pumps oxygenated blood to your muscles, adjusting its pace and volume based on your body's needs. This demonstrates its adaptability and strength. The initial movement and acceleration of the body involve the heart and at least three energy channels. The brain sends wireless and electrical impulses as commands to the lungs, the triple energizer, and the gallbladder channels prompting them to respond to the impulses and to energize the muscles. When you start running, additional energy channels, such as the liver and brain channels, must also work together to sustain the motion.

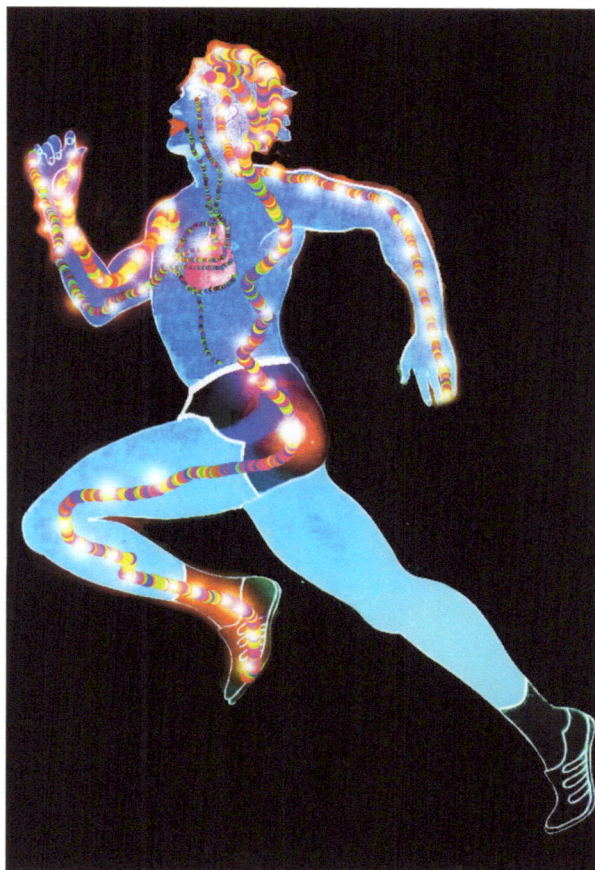

Picture 8. The cooperation of four energy channels at the start of a run.
Own work.

Each movement is initiated by the heart, which provides immediate energy and blood supply to the muscles.

The energy channels included in this particular example of motion are as follows:

- Heart energy channel located on the right arm.
- Lung energy channel runs from below the chest to the thumb of the right arm.
- Triple energizer channel that begins at the fourth finger and ends above the eyebrow.
- The gall bladder channel that runs on the left side of the body from the foot to the head.

The upcoming chapters will explore 10 levels of intelligence within your heart that significantly influence your performance, overall harmony, and physical well-being. Detailed explanations about these levels will be provided in the following chapters.

- Heart's mechanical precision
- Heart's acoustic messaging
- Heart's electromagnetic function
- Heart's neuronal intelligence
- Heart's genomic smartness (DNA)
- Heart's hormonal dominance
- Heart's regenerative power
- Heart's metabolic flexibility
- Heart's quantum connection to the fabric of the Universe
- Heart's emotional intelligence

8

Heart's mechanical precision

Your heart is a phenomenal self-organizing machine that coordinates blood supply throughout the entire body. It has an array of mechanical sensors that detect impulses related to blood circulation and regulate its smooth flow. The sensors, called receptors, are primarily located in the blood vessels and your heart's internal walls. They instantly detect turbulent or vortex flow inside your four heart cavities. They also monitor oxygen saturation, water, minerals in the blood, and blood pressure levels. Other receptors calibrate the volume and temperature of circulating blood according to the body's requirements. Other sensors adjust the body's pH level and monitor mineral balance. When your receptors detect something abnormal, they send signals to release certain hormones from the heart to prevent negative impacts and to restore the natural equilibrium.

Your heart strives for perfection at all times. It can effortlessly rebalance the turbulent vortex flow produced by a temporarily rigid heart wall. Your heart can prevent premature ventricular beats from disturbing and disrupting your smooth blood flow. It maintains a harmonious, smooth rhythm, gentle pulse, and harmonious pressure waves propagating all over the body. Your heart has endurance and can generate a regular heartbeat without a break for an average life span of about 90 to 100 years. Every heartbeat generates a heartbeat-evoked electrical potential in your brain, which travels as an impulse from the brain to the spine and through the nervous system, reaching the entire body. Your cells constantly receive this information from your heart. The downstream flow of this information activates the cells' 7TM receptors and ultimately affects your DNA.

The heart is more than a physical organ; it also generates your emotions. It has messengers called messenger RNA, or mRNA. These molecules stimulate the production of hormones related to your feelings and emotions. This stream of information creates a cascade of living and pulsating information which begins afresh with every heartbeat.

9

Heart's acoustic messaging

Sounds are everywhere in your environment. In modern life, sounds exercise intense power all over your body. It is usually for you to recognize them, assume their origin, or decode the source. However, it takes more sensitivity to recognize sounds coming from inside of your body.

The loudest bodily sound is the breath, the sound of your lungs. The tone of the heartbeat is gentler. But sometimes, paced by anxiety or exertion, the heart can pound loudly.

Fascinating research shows that even stem cell production may respond to acoustic low-frequency signals produced by the heart's sounds. These gentle sounds also affect hormone production, tissue regeneration, the breathing mechanism, and the functioning of the cardiovascular system. The bells of the heart resound in all cells and their DNA, setting off a cascade of life-sustaining signals.

10

Heart's electromagnetic intelligence

Your body contains vibrating and continuously charging atoms and subatomic particles, just like everything else. This electromagnetic reality is basic physics, but it's important to be aware of the electromagnetic nature of the human body when considering your health. The electrically charged particles that make up your body create an invisible but powerful electromagnetic field surrounding you.

The atoms and subatomic particles vibrate at a specific frequency, which is the unique signature of your "quantum existence."

The HeartMath Institute of Research Centre in California, USA, has conducted groundbreaking research confirming the existence of the body's electromagnetic field. This invisible extension of you exchanges information wirelessly within your body and with the external environment. The heart and brain, with their sophisticated systems and bio-computing power, are the primary architects of your magnetic body field. They can transform vast amounts of data into intelligent life-giving information, which is truly awe-inspiring.

11

Heart's neuronal level of intelligence

Your heart and brain are the two most powerful organs, typically working in precise harmony for your well-being. They create coherence and determine your intellectual wellness. When your heart and brain have perfect communication, it can elevate your natural mind to its highest potential.

Your heart also has its own brain, as the contemporary research from 2021 published in the Journal Open Access shows that the heart contains specific neuronal tissue known as "a little brain at the heart."

A perfectly functioning heart is the ultimate safeguard of your general health. The intelligent heart exercises its supreme intelligence in two ways: it uses its own fully independent nervous system and can release specific hormones to calibrate the blood supply to your brain and other internal organs.

12

Heart's genomic wisdom (DNA)

Your heart's genomic wisdom secures long-lasting endurance and optimal functioning of your body. Heart's genes can sustain your heartbeat for 90 up to 100 years. An analysis of all genes shows that the heart has enormous expression of the genes and that the messengers of mRNA are expressed in the heart significantly more than in other internal organs.

It's fascinating that out of the three billion letters that form the entire human genome, only a very small portion (1/60,000 of the entire genome) is unique to us humans. This small fraction is known as the human accelerated regions (HARs), and it sets the human genome apart from all other animals.

Professor Katherine Pollard from the University of California in San Francisco, USA, was the first scientist to discover and describe human accelerated regions (HARs) in 2006.

One of the HARs, the CLOCK gene, aptly named 'circadian locomotors outcome cycles kaput', empowers your heart to overcome any energetic obstruction. The CLOCK gene is a marvel of nature, designed for highly distressing situations to conserve energy resources. It can down-regulate energy production throughout your body and prepare your heart for more critical situations. Activation of this energy negative loop may make you feel powerless and lacking energy. However, in these moments, the stored energy in your body can be instantly released and allows you to perform extraordinary feats. You may recall situations and instances where you surpassed your physical and intellectual capacity. Suddenly, at the brink of life and death, you could conquer extraordinary, life-threatening circumstances. It was your CLOCK gene, a true hero, acting in your heart.

After this extraordinary performance, the heart's CLOCK gene usually returns to regular operation. The return of the positive energy feedback loop restores calmness, allowing you to forget the life-threatening storm.

Recent studies have shown that traumatic experiences in previous generations, such as stress, famine, or war, can deeply impact the expression of your genes. These transmitted traumas, often referred to as intergenerational trauma, can influence which genes are activated or deactivated. Sometimes, a particular situation can trigger emotional and physical responses in your body. Your impulsive reactions may stem from intergenerational "junk" DNA, a term used to describe non-coding DNA. Japanese researchers discovered this DNA in the early 1950s, and while it was initially thought to be functionless, it is now believed to have regulatory roles, acting as DNA software that may affect your temperament. When you are born, you inherit a dominant set of genes from your ancestors, but it is also possible to create your own brand-new DNA. This is why energy channel and awareness training are vital. This concept is known as epigenetics, which is above and dominant over genetics. The newly acquired, brand-new part of your genes becomes more crucial when you engage in physical and spiritual training. When it merges with the dominant intergenerational 'junk' DNA, it can overwrite it and change your responses. Epigenetics acquired in physical and spiritual training plays a significant role in shaping your new personality.

13

Heart's hormonal dominance

The heart's hormones play a key role in the body's hormonal regulation. The four hormones your heart generates every 24 to 48 minutes are not just about metabolism and energy production. They are the guardians of our bodily functions, influencing the stress response, fat metabolism, blood acidity/alkalinity, tissue oxygenation equilibrium, and water/minerals balance.

Your intelligent heart produces four major independent hormones: the atrial natriuretic peptide type A, brain natriuretic peptide type B, first discovered in the brain; type C, first extracted from salmon; and type D. The last one is a close relative of a hormone found in the green mamba.

Your fifth heart's hormone accelerates the energy production of adenosine triphosphate (ATP) to fuel cellular breathing. Your oxygen intake boosts the output of the high-energy ATP available for all cells in your body.

In emergencies when the blood supply to your heart is too low, your heart can produce two additional hormones: cardiomyosin and serum response factor. In such situations, these hormones released by the heart limit the blood supply to the brain when it becomes selfish and demands excessive blood and energy at the expense of other internal organs.

14

Heart's regenerative power

Your heart, a wonder of nature, beats tirelessly for over 90 or even 100 years, necessitating continuous and robust regeneration. A pivotal moment in our understanding of this process came in 2010, when Harvard University unveiled a startling revelation that every hart including your heart, at all times, is actively producing adult omnipotent stem cells. These cells enure the heart's lifelong activity and are the key to regenerating and restoring damaged heart tissue.

The discovery of heart stem cells was a groundbreaking advancement in regenerative medicine. It sparked extensive research into stem cells. Scientific evidence suggests that all internal organs have similar regenerative potential. In 2012, the Nobel Prize was awarded to John B. Gurdon and Dr. Shinya Yamanaka for their work in reprogramming ordinary cells into stem cells that can regenerate all internal organs of the human body. The ability of organs like the liver, kidney, and spleen to produce adult omnipotent stem cells is crucial for the body's lifelong renewal capacity. This research also revealed that even slow-regenerating organs such as the heart (which takes about 20 years for complete renewal) and the brain (which requires approximately 40 years to exchange all neurons and nerve cells) have the potential to fully heal. This means that the body is capable of creating multiple hearts and brains throughout a person's life. The heart plays a central role in the body's self-organizing system. Prolonged stress can lead to adverse changes in the heart, such as enlargement and increased fibrous wall structures. Your heart has the ability to reverse these changes and accomplish positive remodeling within a few months.

The beautiful description of the stem cell can be found in the book *Life and Teachings of the Masters of the Far East* by Baird Spalding published in 1991:

"As the cell divides and creates a new cell, our thought is implanted upon it...In the first cell, all is perfect. That cell was first known as the Christ cell." (i.e., the anointed cell) "It is always just as young as ever it was. It never takes on old age. It is the primal spark of life. When we implant in it our thoughts of limitation or old age, or any condition outside of perfection, the body responds. Cells born from the first cell take on its image. Originally it is the image and likeness of God. It is perfect in every way. But it becomes the form we carry in our minds...if we carry the image of perfection always, what will it do for these cells? It will build perfection." (Vol. 6, Page 78)

15

Heart's metabolic flexibility

The adult heart's metabolic flexibility allows it to switch between different energy sources.

Imagine that your heart has a genetic switch between two engines. One operates when there is an abundance of oxygen, and the other kicks in when your blood has poor oxygenation. The first is called "adult metabolism," and the second is known as "fetal" metabolism.

Adult metabolism is 17 times more efficient in producing energy than fetal metabolism, and it is the natural regulator of the blood supply to the brain.

The fetal metabolic engine is a remnant from your early development in the womb, and it is relevant in emergency situations where, for some reason, you stop breathing. For example, when you hold your breath for a couple of minutes, carbon dioxide retention causes the brain's blood vessels to open maximally, leading to a feeling of euphoria.

This activates the "fetal" metabolism, which primarily burns glucose in response to the oxygen emergency. This is similar to the situation of an unborn fetus because the lungs are not yet working in the womb.

Holding your breath for extended periods can cause headaches, drowsiness, confusion, global transient amnesia, elevated blood pressure, and arrhythmias. Holding your breath longer produces a further increase in carbon dioxide, which can lead to a situation similar to dying.

The adult metabolic engine starts working after your birth. It is activated through emerging function of your lungs in an environment abundant with oxygen. It burns fat instead of glucose. Your heart has the ability to switch between fetal and adult metabolism. This switch is controlled by the PPARγ gene, the peroxisome proliferator-activated receptor. When there is a lack of oxygen in the heart, it signals for the energy production to switch back to the "fetal" inefficient glucose metabolic engine to survive the poor oxygenation.

Your heart can protect you from getting a heart attack by hibernating the heart muscle known also as "hibernating myocardium" in medical language. It reduces metabolism and the blood supply to the affected heart area to the survival level. At the same time, the heart produces a gene, hypoxia-induced factor to adapt the affected heart to low oxygen levels. The hypoxia gene is always triggered through an oxygen emergency It helps protect and sustain hibernating myocardium as long as possible until the oxygen supply returns to normal. Hibernation can continue for a short or long time. It can last minutes, hours, days, months, or even years.

16

Heart's quantum connection to the fabric of the Universe

The quantum connection of the heart refers to its relationship with the invisible world of sub-atomic particles and the unlimited potentiality waves, which together constitute the fabric of the Universe. Generally speaking it refers to your spirituality. Throughout history, the heart has been considered a place of love, compassion, intuition, and wisdom. The heart was, is, and will be a gateway to consciousness, truth, and a spiritual connection with the unseen world.

The HeartMath Institute in California, USA, performed experiments on coherent heart/brain interactions, showing that the human heart contains a specific electromagnetic, wireless connection to the electromagnetic fields around you. In this exciting study, the computers measured an examined person's heart and brain electromagnetic waves. Devices registered both the heart's and the brain's electromagnetic response. The subject sat in front of a screen. The researchers projected randomly pleasant and terrifying images. Amazingly, the heart responded first, and the reaction of the heart was even more stunning; it decoded the images before they appeared on the screen.

This unique ability of your heart sometimes allows you to anticipate future events in a way that surpasses the capabilities of your five senses and the brain's perception. On the other hand, when the heart and brain are not in sync, it can lead to poor concentration, memory, and intellectual discomfort.

17

Heart's emotional intelligence

Emotional intelligence (EI) is the capacity to understand and manage emotions. It allows you to recognize and interpret your own emotions and those of others. Your feelings are a reflection of the world around you, and when you are in a positive state of mind, the fabric of the Universe responds by creating good feelings in you. EI is crucial for social interactions and your connection with the world. It operates at the intersection of consciousness and awareness, and it can function in both physical and spiritual dimensions. Love is the ultimate expression of emotional intelligence, granting you access to the boundless potential of the Universe. Therefore, your heart constantly balances the influence of your brand new, love-based DNA with old, habitual impulses originated from the generational "junk" DNA.

You can excel in your knowledge about your heart's intelligence from the medical perspective by reading my previous book: *"Dyczynski Program. Healing of the intelligent heart"*. It was published in 2021.

18

Brain energy channel. Your smart brain and its mind.

Your brain, a marvel of nature, exerts centralized control over all your internal organs except your heart. It internally weaves a connection to all of your body's energy channels. The brain energy channel is the most complex channel in your body and consists of two energy vessels. One energy vessel, referred to in traditional medicine as the "conception vessel," runs in front of the body. The second, known in natural medicine as the "governing vessel," runs alongside the spine and head. Both energy vessels are linked through the lips, mouth, and tongue.

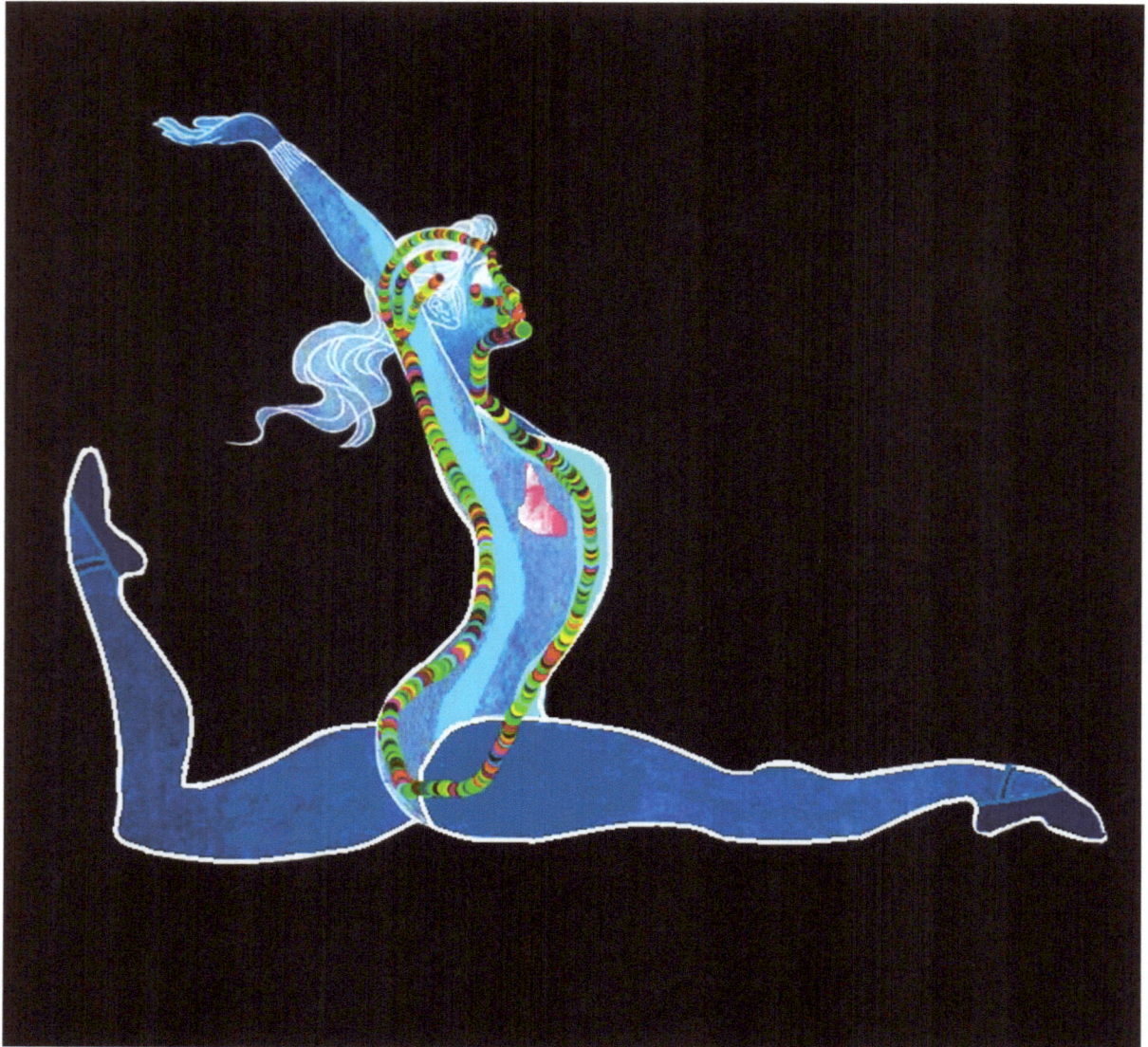

Picture 9. The course of the brain energy channel.
Own work.

Your body responds to your brain's commands, triggering the secretion of beneficial chemicals and hormones and meticulously recording the old and new patterns of your muscle activity. This efficient brain plasticity allows you to adapt to environmental changes. While some basic types of responsiveness, such as reflexes, can be mediated by the spinal cord, solar plexus, or pelvic plexus, it is your brain's task to ensure your correct behavioural response to all sensory and motoric impulses.

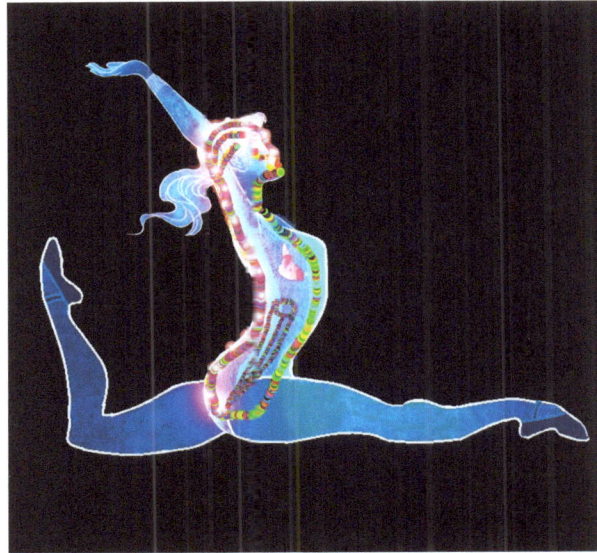

Picture 10. The back part of the brain's energy channel is called the "governing vessel," and its entry points are marked with light. The "governing vessel" originates in the middle abdomen within the solar plexus, and it has internal branches.
Own work.

The back energy vesel, known in traditional medicine as the "governing vessel," starts in the middle abdomen within the solar plexus and emerges from the inside to the outside of the body at the crotch. It then runs from the tip of the spine in the lower back, ascends alongside the entire spine to the neck, enters the brain, and ends at the upper lip.

The front energy vessel of the brain channels, referred to in natural medicine as the "conception vessel," forms its flow in the middle line of the front of your body.

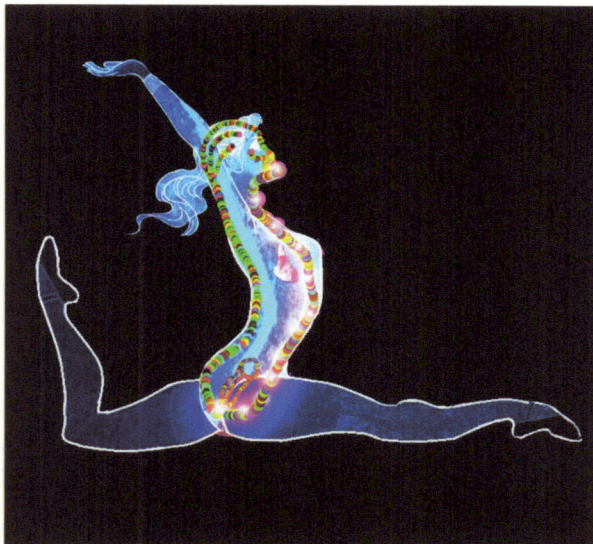

Picture 11. The front part of the brain energy channel is known as the "conception vessel," with its entry points marked with light. The origin area of the "conception vessel," with its internal branches inside the lower abdomen, within the pelvic plexus, is also displayed.
Own work.

It originates inside the lower abdomen within the pelvic plexus, breaks out to the outside of the body at the crotch (the small area between the end of the bowel and the reproductive organs), ascends to the front of your body, connects to the reproductive organs and the heart, and ends at the lower lip. These two energy vessels form the brain energy channel and work together to circulate energy during your orbital breathing.

Modern neuroscience is fascinated by the way your brain and its software mind work. Your brain operates as a biological computer, but its processes are different from those of a digital computer. It acquires, stores, and processes information from the surrounding world using quantum bits. This unique feature enables it to perform millions of operations simultaneously in the same or different areas of your brain.

The below-listed levels of your brain's smartness specifically influence your bodily harmony and intellectual well-being. Their more detailed description is presented in the following chapters:

- Your thinking and reasoning
- Your mind's healing capability
- The miniaturized representation of your body in the brain
- The mirror neurons in your brain
- The dormant brain
- Your potential to change the dormant brain

19

Your thinking and reasoning

Remember these crucial facts about your brain while thinking and reasoning and making your training. Your brain consists of delicate tissue, and it is essential to life. It needs to be well-protected, as it is encased in layers of bone and immersed in nourishing fluid.

According to US researcher VanWeeden of Massachusetts General Hospital in Boston, the brain has a perfect geometric, three-dimensional structure. This was based on a study conducted in 2011 using Magnetic Resonance Imaging. The brain organizes itself like a street grid in cities such as Perth or New York City. It is no surprise that the brain, governing the divine geometry of your body and its perfect symmetry, is itself very well organized.

The fluid in the brain and its extension, the spine, moves uniquely in a "cerebrospinal rhythm," mimicking dolphins in a swimming rhythm. Your brain is made up of two hemispheres, each with specialized functions, known as lateralization, which differentiates the left and right brain.

Your brain, a powerhouse of energy, is intimately connected to your heart. It relies entirely on the blood supply from it. Your brain controls the chain block for metabolism and energy production utilizing a lot of energy in form of glucose and oxygen. In fact, it consumes about 200 g of sugar daily or 73 kg annually, testifying its constant demand for high energy fuel. Take a look at the image below. It's a glimpse into the web of interconnections within your brain. This is a complex computer-like network. It makes your brain such a fascinating and highly sophisticated organ.

Your brain is a remarkable organ, responsible for your thinking, intellect, and reasoning. Second only to the heart, it serves as the crucial link between your body and the world around you. Your mind acts as a sophisticated software application, facilitating the exchange of vital information between your brain and heart, effectively integrating your body with the external environment, through the energy channels.

20

Your mind's healing capability

From that time Jesus began to preach and say" Turn to God and change the way you think and act, because the kingdom of heaven is near " Matthew 3, Verse 2

Since 2008, extensive research has been dedicated to establishing evidence for the effectiveness of mind-body interventions and mind-body medicine. The US National Center for Complementary and Integrative Health defines mind-body interventions as activities that purposefully affect mental and physical fitness, listing activities such as yoga, tai chi, Pilates, guided imagery, guided meditation and forms of meditative praxis, hypnosis, hypnotherapy, and prayer, as well as art therapy, music therapy, and dance therapy.

The mind-body medicine is centered on exploring the connections between the brain, mind, body, and behavior, and their profound impact on overall health, healing and wellness.

Recently, the medical research and scientists have found solid evidence that mind body techniques do strengthen the immune system, do fight the illness and promote health.

Your brain and its software mind are equipped with numerous "apps" that automatically perform vital functions crucial to life. Additionally, the brain weaves the body's energy channels, connecting them to the circular energy flow of orbital breathing.

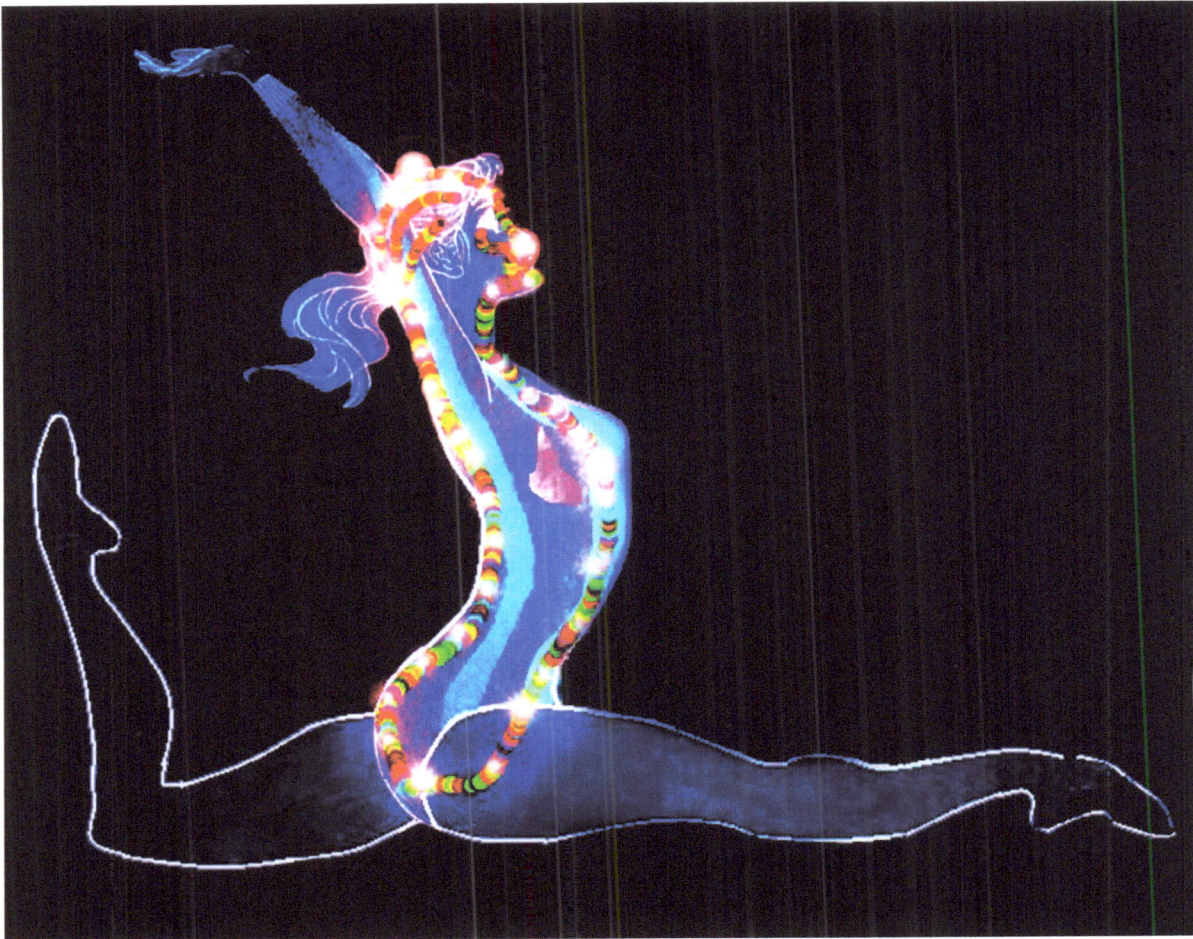

Picturde 12. The course of the brain energy channel. The entry points marked with light.
Own work.

As the ultimate supervisor, your mind plays a pivotal role in your health and healing, controlling intelligence, wisdom, beliefs, desires, intentions, and emotions. It acts as a master conductor, overseeing bodily functions to balance and coordinate activities being at your will-power. Brain translates these wireless commands and sends out electrical impulses that prompt your, breathing to accelerate, your muscles to contract, relax, or to move.

Your mind issues commands to your lungs, directing them to take deeper breaths. Diaphragmatic and orbital breathing enhance venous return to your heart. This leads to increase of the blood volume generated by your heart. In turn it results in better blood supply to your brain and other internal organs. Your focused attention on the energy flow during orbital breathing and on your brain energy channel will empower the functionality of your brain.

21

The mini representation of the body in the brain for your healing

Did you know that your body and brain form an incredible self-organizing system? Your brain contains a detailed map of your entire body, with each side of your brain controlling the opposite side of your body. This internal map serves as a blueprint for the mind and DNA to guide healing and restore functionality when the body is injured or needs repair. Tissue regeneration, wound healing, and restoring lost functions all follow this amazing internal bodily plan.

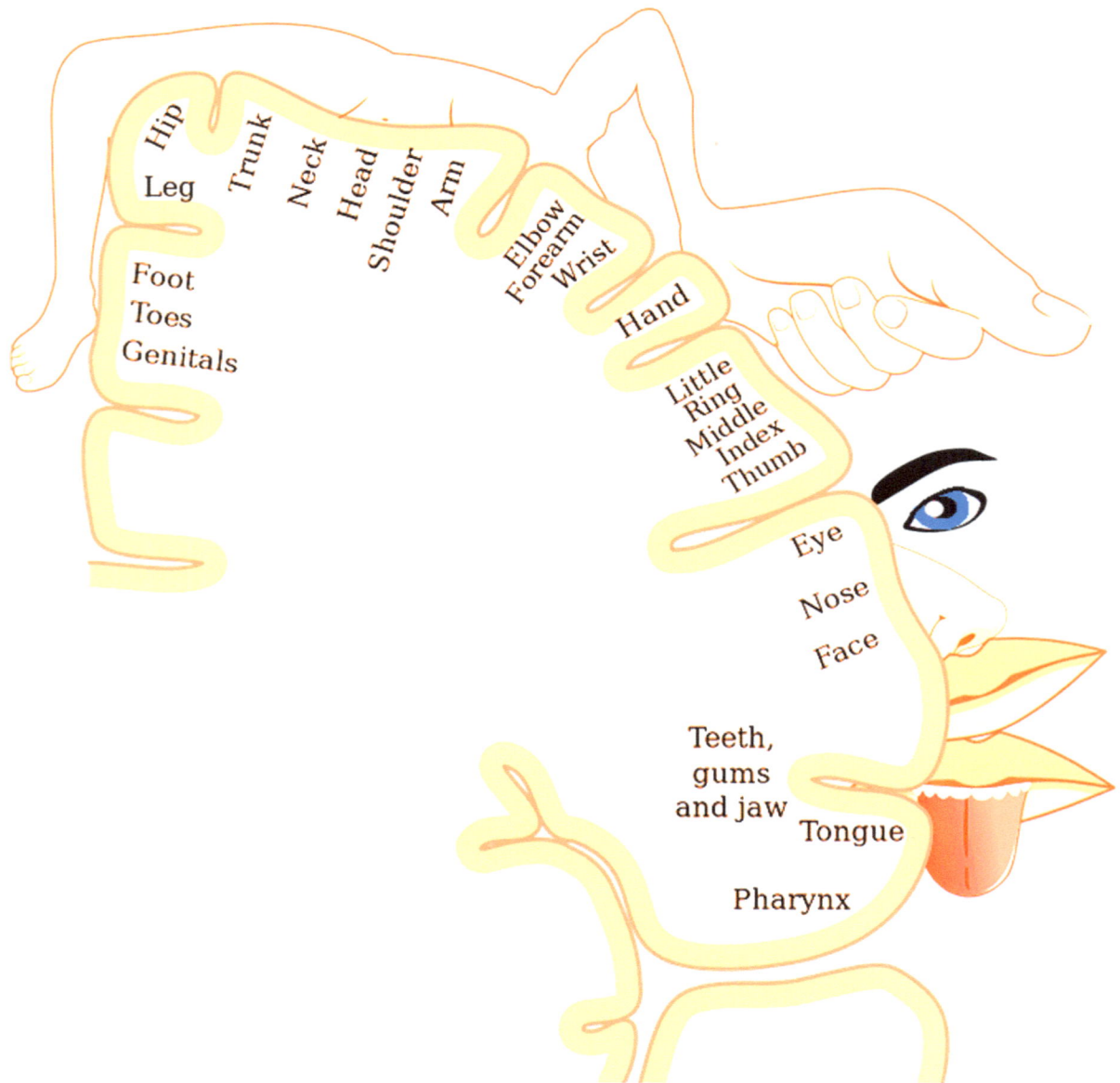

Picture 13. The homunculus, the representation of the body in the brain.

Your brain is also very specialized and diversified in its functionality. This is known as a lateralization. The lateralization of your brain function is the tendency for some brain functions or visual processing of the data to be specialized to one side of the brain or the other.

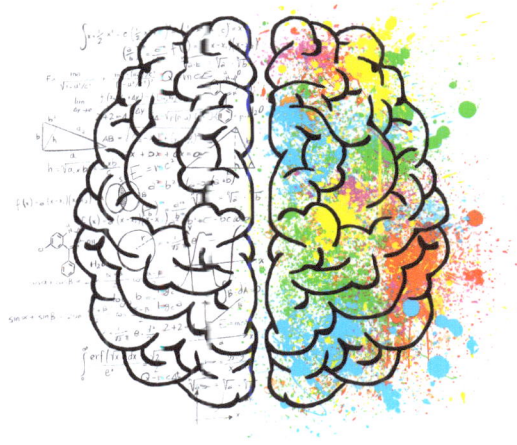

Picture 14. The left side of the brain is more for numbers, mathematics, and logical thinking, and the right is more for images, colors, and art.
By ElisaRiva - https://pixabay.com/en/ brain-mind-psychology-idea-drawing-2062057/ archive copy, CC0, https://commons.wikimedia.org/w/ index.php?curid=75737264

Therefore, due to lateralization of your brain, you will train to sequentially engage the left and right parts of your body, stimulating an identical pattern in your brain. This method is essential for maintaining the harmonious balance between the right and left parts of your brain.

22

The dormant brain

Your brain needs energy, blood, oxygen, and essential nutrients to function with excellence. Your heart supplies the brain 24/7 by pumping fresh blood into it with every heartbeat. The mechanical pulse and pressure waves produced by each heartbeat create the brain's electrical response, which spreads throughout your body. This is a part of the internal communication between your heart and brain. When certain areas of your brain experience a temporary lack of blood and oxygen supply, it is a cause for concern for your neurons, the building blocks of your brain. They can die or be saved by entering a dormant state. While in this state these neurons are not functioning optimally, the low functionality keeps them alive.

Dormant brains can lead to sluggish functionality, reduced energy, impaired memory, and clouded thinking. Prolonged inactivity can cause low vitality and even depression. If you are experiencing these symptoms, it is wise to consider rebalancing your heart and brain.

This dormant state of your brain can accelerate the aging of neurons and impair the brain's ability to regenerate and rewire itself. However, there is a positive aspect: you can revive your brain cells , reverse these troubling symptoms and improve your memory.

Surprisingly, the root cause may not be in your brain but in your heart, which may be in a state of hibernation, failing to deliver sufficient blood and oxygen to your brain.

Your heart due to distress, lack of oxygen, emotional traumas, or a spasm of your coronary artery can go into hibernation prior to brain dormancy. Your dysfunctional heart will reduce the blood supply to your brain.

This mismatched blood supply between the heart and brain affects the energy flow in the body's energy channels, leading to tiredness and feelings of low-level energy.

It is important to understand that the interactions between opposing forces in this situation can be unpredictable if not addressed through intensified self-observation and appropriate action. Understanding and regulating this dynamic within your body can prompt you to take proactive steps toward maintaining your heart and brain health.

23

The mirror neurons in your brain

Little did we know that the brain houses a unique cell known as mirror neurons. Their discovery and research established that they are helpful in learning and mimicking, particularly in visual learning. However, this great discovery was not the outcome of a meticulously planned experiment. Instead, the researchers discovered the mirror neurons in a simple accident. In the early 1980s, a team of Italian researchers from the University of Parma, led by Dr. Giacomo Rizolatti, were studying the reactions in monkeys' brains to food. The monkey had finished eating and closely watched the scientist who was preparing for the next experiment. In the moment the researcher instinctively grabbed nuts from a bowl the monkey's brain showed the same firing activity as when it had eaten the nuts.

This was an electrifying moment, a thrilling discovery in the realm of neuroscience.

Isn't it awesome to have mirror neurons in your brain? Further human experiments confirmed that your brain can produce the same pattern of electrical activity independently of whether you are eating or only observing someone eating.

Billions of people are drawn to watching football or other sports games on television, and it is not just the thrill of the game but also the activation of their mirror neurons. In essence, they are virtually playing football, experiencing the same emotions of victory or defeat as the players on the field.

You are not just a passive observer but an active participant in learning through your mirror neurons. Your mirror neurons fire impulses when you observe others' actions as if you were the one performing them. This is the essence of quantum entanglement. It is a true game-changer to understand your own behaviour fully.

24

Your potential to change the dormant brain

Remember that you are a knowledgeable observer. Do not wait. It is a waste of time. Act now to change your dormant brain. Lie down and start breathing with your diaphragm, visualizing the orbital flow of the energy supplying your brain. If you don't notice improvement, consider consulting your GP or even calling an ambulance.

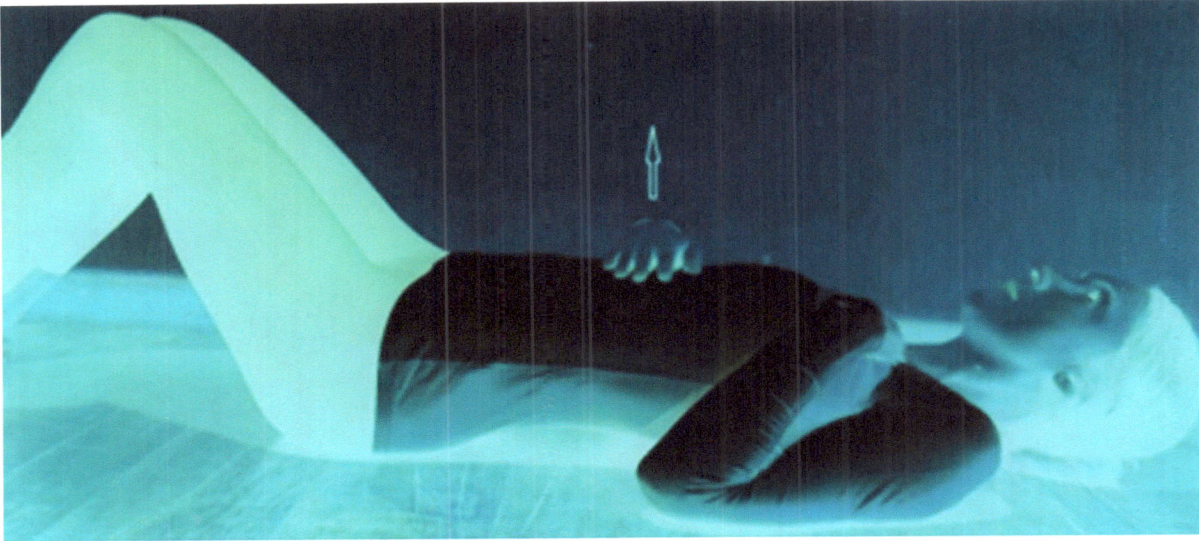

Picture 15. Orbital breathing.
Courtesy of Brittany Giadresco, Nee Ford.

Recognize the power of your intention in this process. By practicing orbital breathing, you can increase the oxygenation and blood supply to your heart and brain, taking a step towards restoring normality. Your brain has the potential to initiate this change. The inspired action with your breathing practice can help you distance yourself from any emotional trauma or distress you may have just experienced.

When you awake your dormant brain cells, you will experience your healing potential first-hand. When you overcame this adverse scenario of your heart and brain, you will feel good again, like nothing has happened to you.

25

Your body's energetic grace

Then, by grace, we present our bodies as instruments of righteousness to God. Romans 6:13

Your body processes a vast amount of information daily, similar to the concept of 'big data' in technology. There are two sources of information: one internal, generated by your heart, mind, soul, and spirit, and the other external, originating from your physical and social environment.

Just as technology utilizes "big data" to make informed decisions, your body uses this information in the best possible way to stay vital, maintaining your good health and mobility.

It is essential to train daily, whether in a gym or outdoors, to build physical endurance and fitness. This effort is rewarding but also challenging. If you aim to achieve bodily grace along with physical fitness, it is important to train smart your body.

Remember that your body has energy channels that interact with the universal law of gravitation and environmental impact. Training these energy channels helps you face daily challenges such as exposure to pollution, toxins, and viruses.

Awareness training will also help you cope with extreme weather changes such as cold or heat day by day. You encounter a gravitational field daily and have overcome physical and mental challenges in your living space.

To maintain flexibility and a vibrant lifestyle, it is beneficial to combine traditional and modern training. Through better understanding the underlying laws for energy wining in those two approaches to training you will harness more vitality. It is like your two lungs which complement each other and are working in perfect harmony. It gives you wings by running. Integrated approach for training can unlock your body's full potential, leading to purposeful and graceful fitness gives you also confidence in your health choices, knowing you are utilizing the best of both worlds.

Your body's motion is a fascinating energy process, of commands from your brain, and a delicate balance of blood and oxygen supply delivered by your intelligent heart to your internal organs and muscles.

Your heart, the conductor of your bodily energy system delivers its complex actions for your best performance. Your brain, the mastermind, supports it entirely when you fully focus on your body and the movements.

Finding the harmony where your nerves, bones, muscles, and ligaments can follow your heart's intelligent work and your brain's innovative activity is a complex task. But remember, your body's potential is infinite, and by understanding and harnessing its energy, you hold the reins for your best performance.

The perspectives on bio-energy in traditional and modern Western medicine are consistent and complementary.

The Western perspective defines 'bio-energy' as the energy generated by metabolism, which is the series of chemical reactions in the body's cells that convert food and oxygen into energy. This energy is essential for bodily functions such as movement, cognition, fighting infections, and growth. The metabolic processes produce energy by converting food and oxygen into adenosine triphosphate (ATP), which is the universal energy carrier in the body.

There are two main pathways for ATP production: one with oxygen and one without. Both pathways utilize glucose as the energy source. The primary system burns oxygen producing a significant amount of ATP. It can sustain your muscle function during intense exercise for about 60 minutes or more.

The secondary system is serving as a backup of energy production in emergency situation, where oxygen is missing. It produces a little amount of ATP and can only sustain intense exercise for less than two minutes.

The primary energy system, which relies on oxygen, requires 550 liters of pure oxygen or 2200 liters of air daily without any exercises. During activities such as running, the primary energy system provides more than 80 percent of the energy for the first kilometer. If the activity continues, your body may reach a point of energy depletion, commonly known as "hitting the wall." To overcome this functional barrier will require from you to increase oxygen intake with your well-trained respiratory system. Though your energy channel training you will be supported by well-ventilated lungs, strong breathing muscles, and a well-trained diaphragm,

It is important to note that the primary and secondary energy systems usually work together, and it is not about one system replacing the other, but rather about their relative dominance during different activities and training.

As you become more aware of your body's energy channels, you will better understand how your mind and muscles can become more efficient at sensing your movement patterns and correcting them promptly. This experience will reveal your potential for self-improvement and develop a holistic awareness of your body. It will inspire and motivate you to strive for better fitness and higher energy levels.

Your pattern of sequential limbs and body movements is unique. It is made naturally or can result from specialized training. Your gait is particular to you due to your daily habits and personal history of traumas, injuries, and illnesses. Your kinetic pattern, a combination of moves, applied muscular force, and contractile speed, is not only influenced by your primary energy system (with oxygen) or the secondary one (without oxygen), but also by your informed choices. Training your energy channels will shape not only how your feet interact with the ground, but also how your body follows the feet, giving you a sense of confidence over your graceful movements.

You can internally decode your patterns of bodily motion and you have a unique sense of detecting movements in your environment. Sensing your self-movement, feeling of applied force, and body position is subtle and requires concentration. The neurons and receptors within muscles, tendons, and joints play an important role in this process. Training them to be more vigilant in your awareness training of energy channels is crucial. Your role in stabilizing body posture and coordinating body movement is not just important; it is essential in understanding the inside of your body.

The perception of motion in your environment is a fascinating phenomenon. It occurs when an object or entity changes its position relative to its surroundings. As an observer, you can identify and interpret the physical movement, changes in location, displacement in time, and alterations in light. For instance, you can recognize a person from far away without seeing their face. You can identify the unique gait or specific movements of the person you know, proving the accuracy of your external perception of motion.

Let's take a look at picture below. In this image, we see three runners in action. The runner in the back and on the far right is in the suspended phase, a moment in the running cycle where neither foot touches the ground. This is a perfect example of external perception of motion, where we can observe and identify the physical movement of the runner.

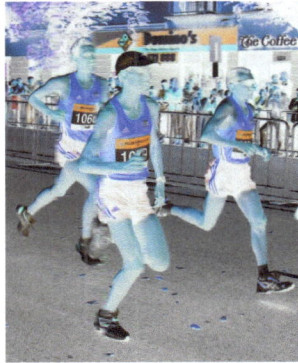

Picture 16. Three runners in action. Reverse colour view.
By Melburnian - Own work, CC BY 2.5https://commons.wikimedia .org/w/ index.php?curid=1420320

You can improve your energy channel exercises by training the sequenced patterns and controlling the speed of your movements. Focus by your moves on contracting and extending slowly your muscles to gain better control over your movements.

26

The six primary energy channels

The six primary internal organs - the heart, brain, liver, spleen, lungs, and kidneys serve as energy powerhouses that produce life energy. These are six energy channels connected to the six primary internal organs:

1. Heart energy channel: including solar plexus/small intestine/pericardium/lymphatic system
2. Brain energy channel: including spinal column/ solar and pelvic plexus/ autonomous system /nervus vagus / the microcosmic orbit related to the breathing mechanism/ magnetic sensing through receptors in the ethmoid bone located between the eyes
3. Spleen energy channel: including /stomach/pancreas/immune system as the parts of the digestive system
4. Lung energy channel: including other parts of the respiratory system /diaphragm/upper airways/ and the large intestine
5. Kidney energy channel: including adrenals/uterus/prostate/reproductive organs/ bladder, as the parts of the reproductive system
6. Liver energy channel: including gallbladder and parts of the hormone system

27

The six supportive energy channels

The six supportive internal organs are:

1. The small intestine supports the heart system
2. The spinal column, solar and pelvic plexus, cranial nerves support the brain system
3. The stomach supports the spleen in the digestive functions
4. The large intestine supports the lungs in the elimination of toxins and wastes
5. The urinary bladder supports the kidneys
6. The gallbladder supports the liver
7. These supportive internal organs have the energy channels, which mainly distribute the energy produced by the six primary organs.

Did you know that there is an additional energy channel related to the pericardium? Pericardium is the protective sac surrounding the heart. This pericardial channel is part of the lymphatic system. Pericardium with its movements reflecting the beating heart influences the lymph nodes and all lymphatic vessels in your body. This unique lymphatic energy channel is intertwined with other energy channels referred to as the triple energizer, which links the lymphatic function of the three essential cavities of your body: the chest, abdomen, and pelvis. The existence of these two additional energy channels is a topic of intense debate in traditional medicine. Some scientists see the lymphatic system as an entity that includes organs like the pericardium, while others believe it should be viewed as a purely functional network.

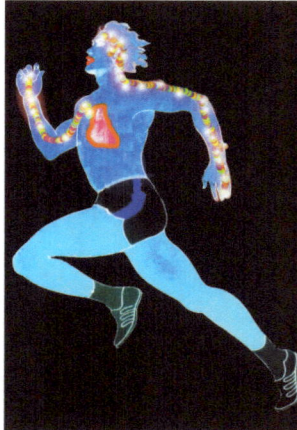

Picture 17. The energy channel of the triple energizer is displayed on the left arm, neck, and head. The course of the pericardium energy channel is marked on the right arm and chest.
Own work.

Both channels belong to the lymphatic system of the body. Pericardium energy channel starts at the chest, one inch beside the nipple and, and ends at the tip of the middle finger. It has 9 entry points marked with light. Triple energizer energy channel starts at the fourth finger and ends at the eyebrow above the eye. It has 23 entry points marked with light. You can memorize the course of the channels and the entry points in your awareness training. The therapists use them for acupuncture or massage.

28

The energy channels training

The energy channel training consists of six postures involving movements of the legs, torso, arms, and hands. It is designed to be easily memorized and repeated. Begin the training by moving the left side of your body, starting with the left leg. After repeating this sequence several times, proceed to the right side of your body, starting with the right leg.

Each training sequence is designed for two complementing each other energy channels.

- heart/small intestine
- brain/spine
- spleen/stomach
- lungs/large intestine
- kidney/urinary bladder
- liver/gall bladder

These particular patterns of moves helps you relax the muscles related to one channel while inducing tension in the muscles associated with another. It creating a balance and harmony that is essential for your good health.

Traditional medicine, which promotes holistic health, emphasizes the importance of muscle relaxation during physical training. The energy channels act as a network of life force, running through your body from the feet to the head and vice versa. The energy channels harmonize functions of the internal organs and connecting you to your direct environment.

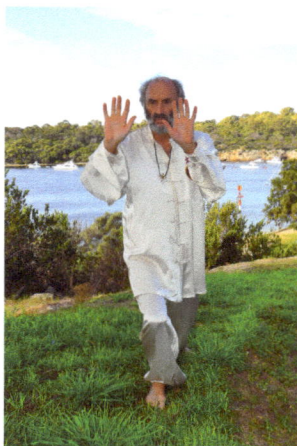

Picture 17. A sequence of training for the liver energy channel.
Own work.

The harmonious teamwork of the energy channels under the supervision of the heart and brain is the essence of holistic health. When every part of your body is mapped in your awareness and connected to the energy channels network, it functions in its optimal mode. This is good for your health and well-being.

29

Heart channel and its energetic training

The heart energy channel is a major player in your body's energetic system. It starts from the heart, located at the centre of your chest. Then it wraps around the heart system to create a powerful vitality network within your body.

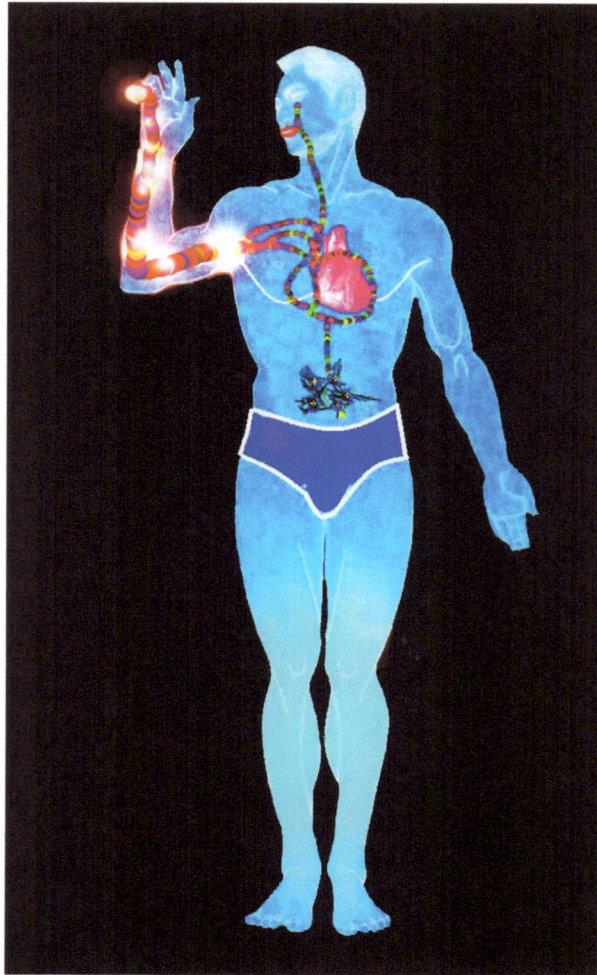

Picture 18. Heart energy channel with its connection to the solar plexus.

The side view of the heart channel. It breaks to outside of your body through the middle of the armpit and proceeds alongside the arm to the last point at the tip of the small finger.

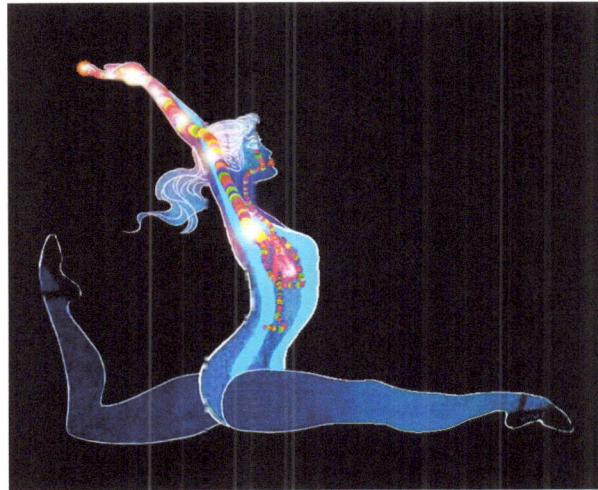

Picture 19. The side view of the heart's energy channel.
The internal branches connect heart energy channel to
the eyes and solar plexus. The gateway points are like
nodes. They are entrances for data and energy
transmission or redistribution.
Own work.

The heart channel has nine entry points marked with light at the following picture. These gateway points can be used for your awareness training. The therapists use them for acupuncture, or massage.

Energetic training for the heart energy channel.

Focus on the heart region in the middle of your chest and the middle of your hands' palms. Please take a stance for the heart's energetic training. Stand upright with a little bit bent knees (soft knee) and face the direction where the sun reaches the highest point, usually south. Your palms, your natural tools to handle the vital energy.

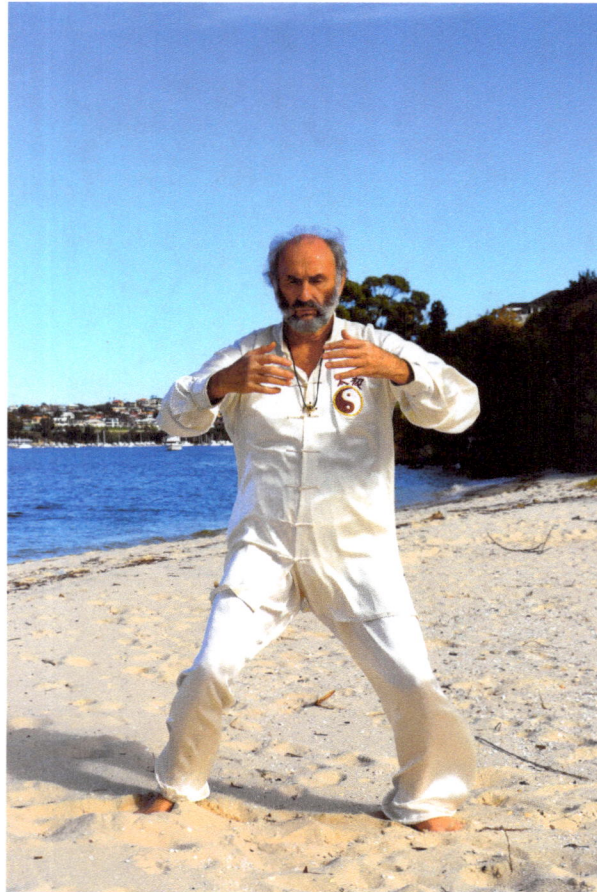

20. Energetic training for the heart channel.
Own work.

Remeber the heart channel starts in the heart, reaches the arms and forearms, and ends at the small finger. This simple yet powerful training puts you in control of your heart energy flow, empowering you to improve your vitality. Now, imagine you're a graceful dancer. Turn your palms outward and with a sweeping motion, move them with your arms in front of your chest about 90 degrees to the left several times and then the same to the right.

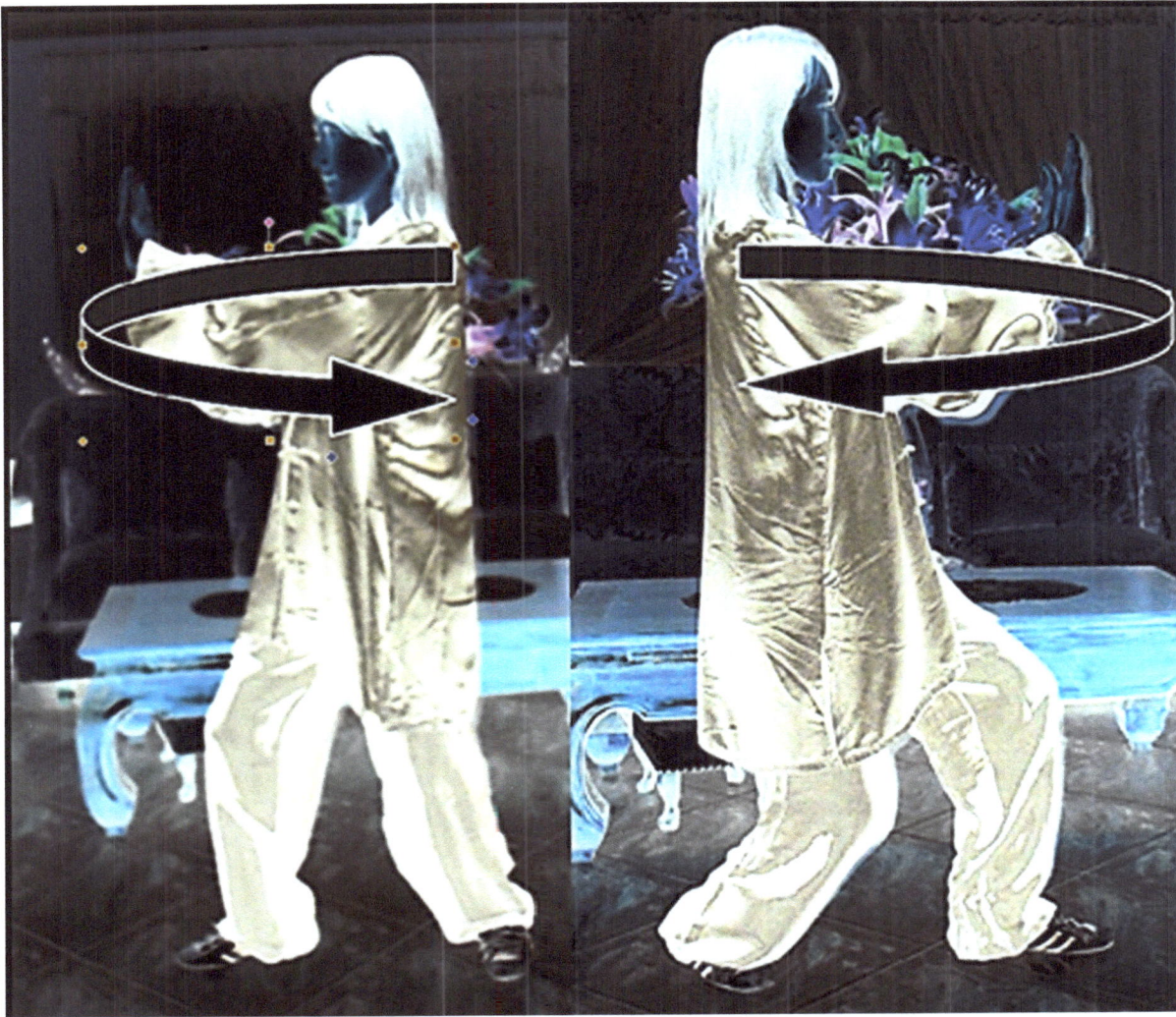

Picture 21. Energetic training for the heart. Semicircular, bow-shaped movement of the open palms and the body. *Own work.*

Please imagine your palms touching the invisible dome around you, the electromagnetic heart field during the rotation in front of the chest.

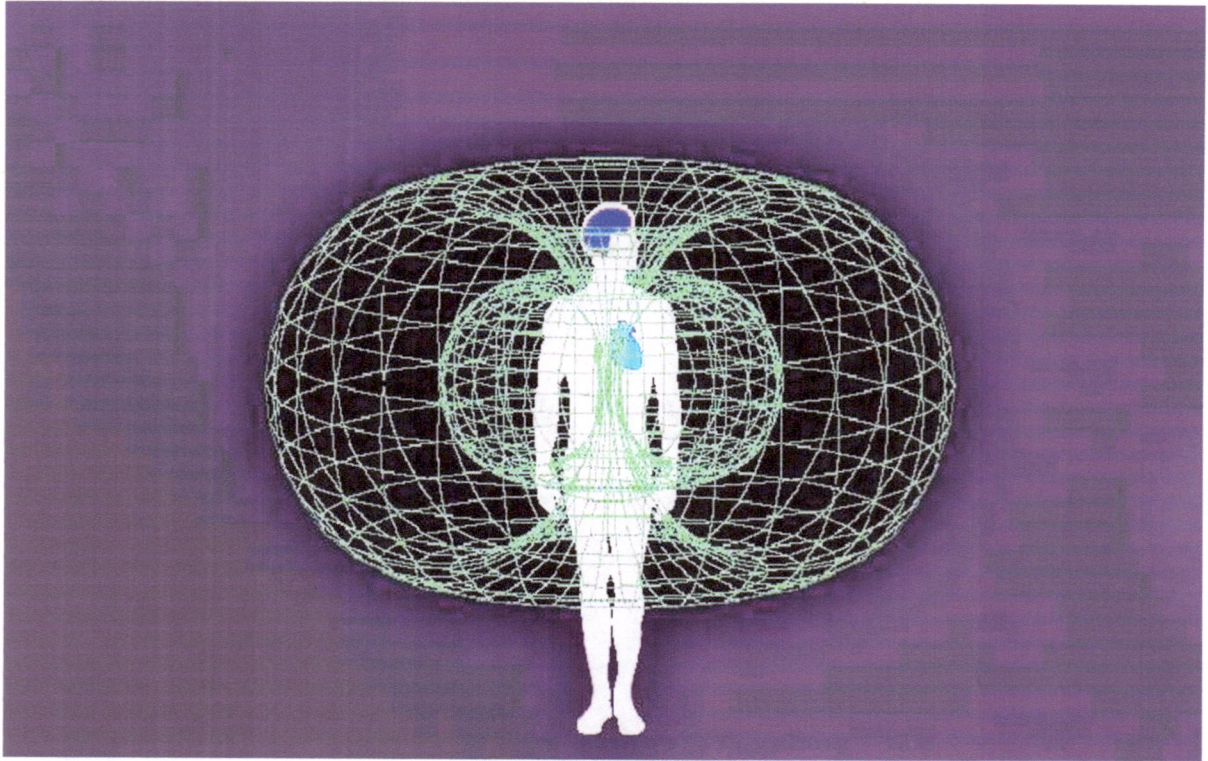

Picture 22. Electromagnetic platform of the human body, particulaly related to the heart and brain.
hearthttps://commons.wikimedia.org/w/index.php?curid=2268503

The small intestine energy channel. It starts at the small finger and ends just below the eye. It has 19 gateway points. It gives two branches to the heart and to the solar plexus.

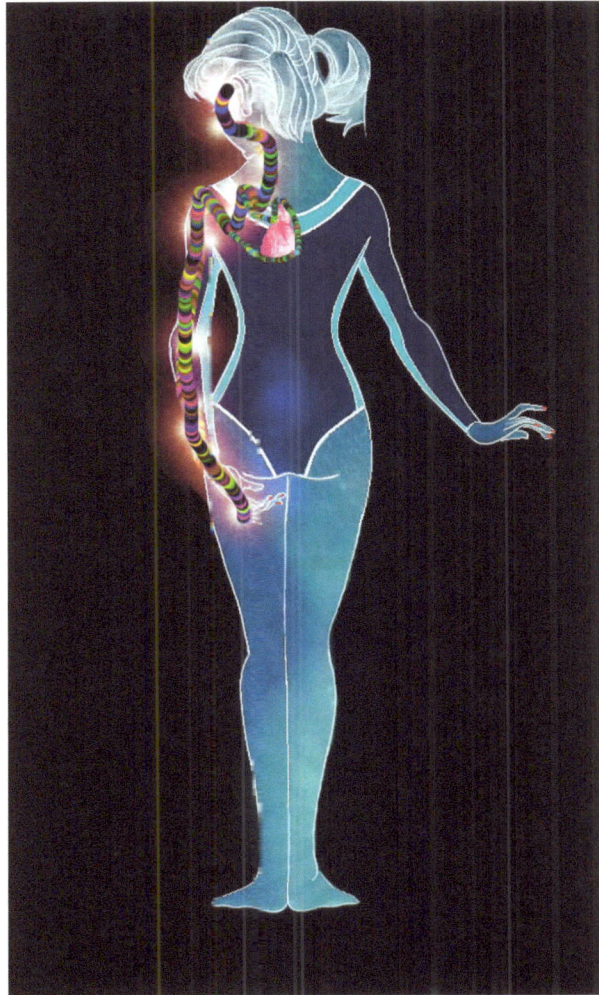

Picture 23. The course of the small intestine energy
channel.
Own work.

30

Brain channel and its energetic training

The brain energy channel, a fundamental component of breathing, exercises, and meditation, it is your gateway to enhanced vitality.

The brain energy channel comprises two traditional medicine energy vessels. The front part of the brain energy channel is called the "conception vessel". It emerges from the perineum (crotch) then it runs through the pelvic region, reproductive organs, abdomen, and chest, and ends at the bottom lip of the mouth.

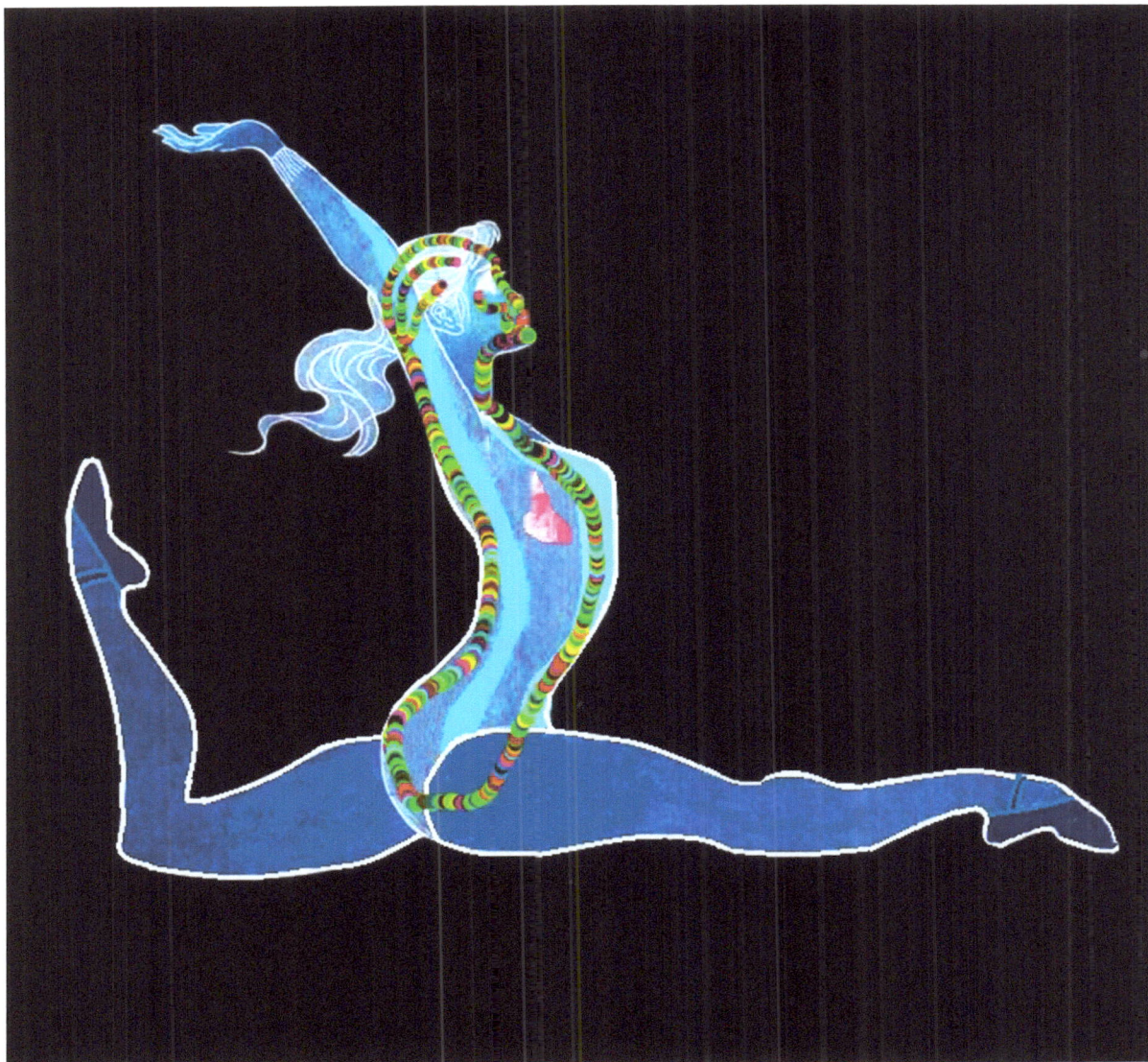

Picture 24. The course of the brain energy channel.
Own work.

The brain energy channel is the platform for vital energy flow during orbital breathing.During each breath, vital energy flows through the brain energy channel. It starts from the lower and middle abdomen within the solar plexus, moves to the groin, and ascends along the spine to reach the skull base, which is known as the "door to the brain." At this point, it enters the brain and then climbs to the highest point of the head, ultimately ending at the entry point between the nose and upper lip.

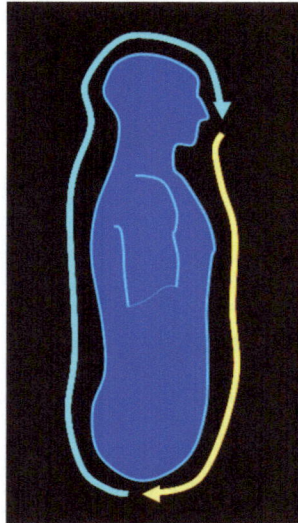

25. Picture. Simplified version of the micro-cosmic orbit.
By Bostjan46 - Own work, CC0.https://commons.wikimedi a.org/w/ index.php?curid=18986673

The front channel of the brain energy, known in traditional medicine as the "conception vessel", originates in the lower abdomen, within the pelvic plexus. Its 24 entry points are marked with light. The front part of the brain energy channel begins inside the lower abdomen, then sends branches downward to the perineum. After that it extends outward at the crotch to the outside of the body. Further it runs along the midline of the front of the body and ends its course at the bottom lip.

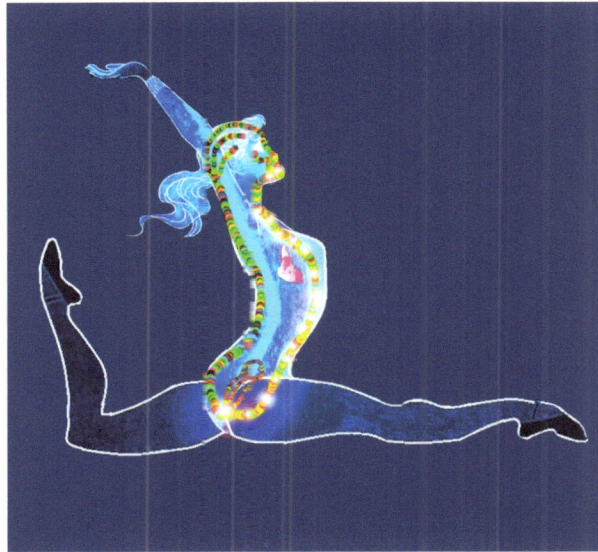

Picture 26. The front "conception vessel" of the brain energy channel.
Own work.

The back part of the brain energy channel, known in traditional medicine as the "governing vessel," starts in the lower and middle abdomen within the solar plexus. It then extends outside the body at the groin area and runs alongside the spine, branching towards the brain at the top of the cervical spine. From there, it ascends to the top of the head and descends to the upper lip. The mouth cavity, the lips and the tongue interconnect the "governing vessel" and the "conception vessel" linking them to the united brain energy channel.

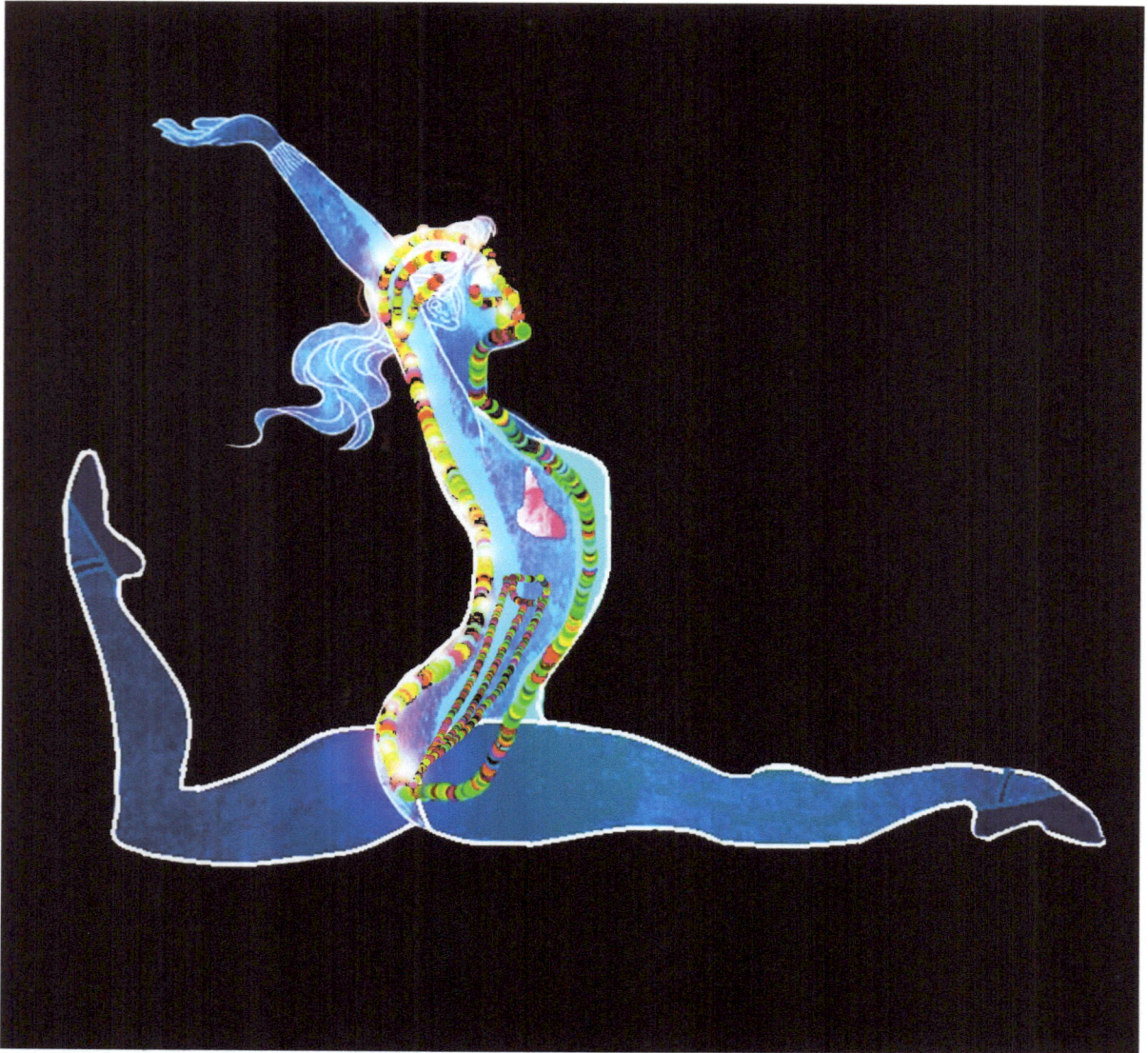

Picture 27. The back part of the brain energy channel, known as the "governing vesel" with its origin within solar plexus.

Own work.

The body's energy channel runs along the front and back, and vital energy circulates between the head and groin. The lips connect the "conception and governing vessel" in one energy channel, closely linked to the breathing mechanism. It's important to undergo awareness training to feel the energy channel and understand the cardinal vital entry points and the flow of energy.

The entry point at the top of the head of the brain's energy channel is very significant in spiritual meaning. It is associated with the energy exchange between your body and the universe. This point is also responsible for the tendons and ligaments that support your body's structure.

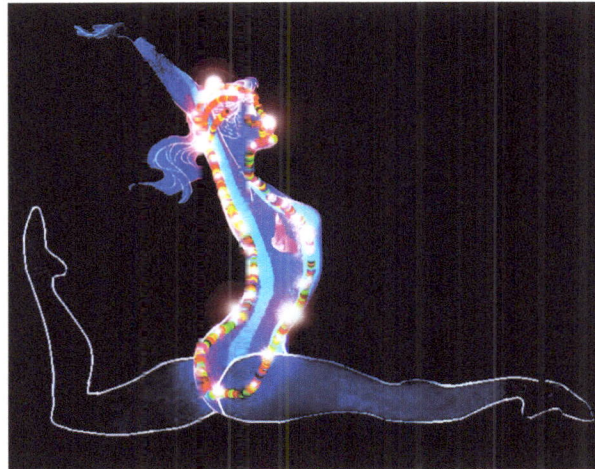

Picture 28. The course of the brain energy channel with
all 51 entry points marked with light.
Own work.

The brain's energy channel begins about two inches below the navel, where breathing originates. In traditional medicine, this point is referred to as "the gate to heaven." The corresponding point on the lower back, at the height of the 5th lumbar vertebra, is called "the gate to life." Both points are considered sources of vitality. The entry point directly under the nose is known as the emergency or revival point, and in common language, it is sometimes called the fear point.

With practice, you can visualize the entire energy channel, elevating your energy to a new level. It helps you to maintain steadiness even during high-performance challenges in modern life.

Energetic training for the brain energy channel.

First, start by gathering vital energy with your hands close to the ground. Then, slowly stand up and move your hands alongside the front part of the brain channel. In the middle of your body, turn your palms around to form a hand prayer gesture, and bring your hands up to your face.

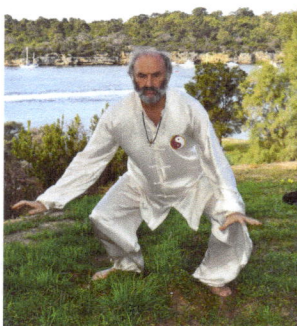

Picture 29. Brain channel training requires gathering energy from the middle of abdomen and assertively moving it upwards along the brain energy channel.
Own work.

Then go higher, just above the highest point of your head, pointing with your thumbs towards the tip of your head. Your attention and your mind focus on the moves. Breathe deeply and consciously. Visualize the energy flowing from the base of your spine to your head and upper lip as you inhale.

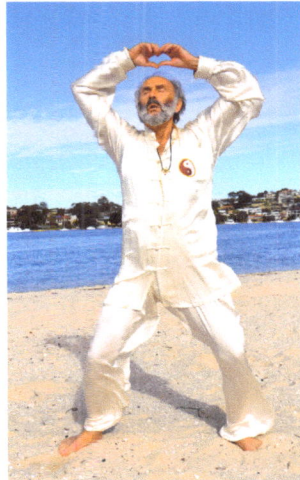

Picture 30. Energetic training of the brain channel.
Own work.

Hold your breath for a moment before exhaling and directing the energy from your lower lip to your lower abdomen and crotch. Then release the energy putting your arms vigorously down. At the same time lower your arms in the bow-like movement and go down with your body reaching the initial position displayed in the picture above. Repeat the sequence several times.

31

Spleen channel and its energetic training

The spleen energy channel starts at the tip of the big toe, runs upwards inside the leg and thigh to the pelvic region close to the reproductive organs, and then goes up on the belly connecting to your spleen, and runs to the side of the chest, where it enters the chest space. It has two internal branches. One brunch goes to the mouth and lips and the other to the heart. The spleen channel has 21 gateway points you can memorize for your awareness training. The therapists use these entry points for treatment with acupuncture or massage.

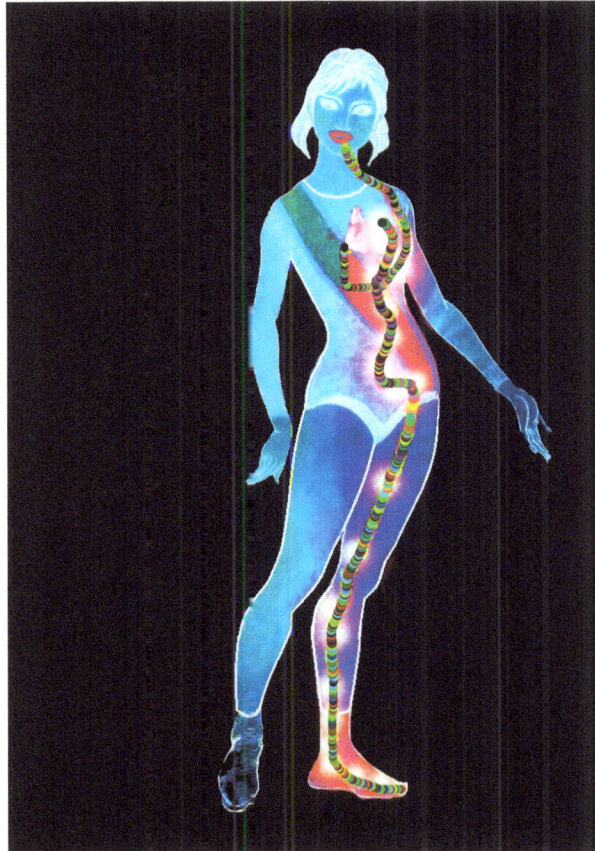

Picture 31. The course of the spleen energy channel.
Own work.

Energetic training for the spleen energy channel.

Step with your left foot forward, facing the sky where the sun reaches the highest point, usually the south, and balance most of your weight on it. Focus on the spleen and stomach on the left side under the ribcage.

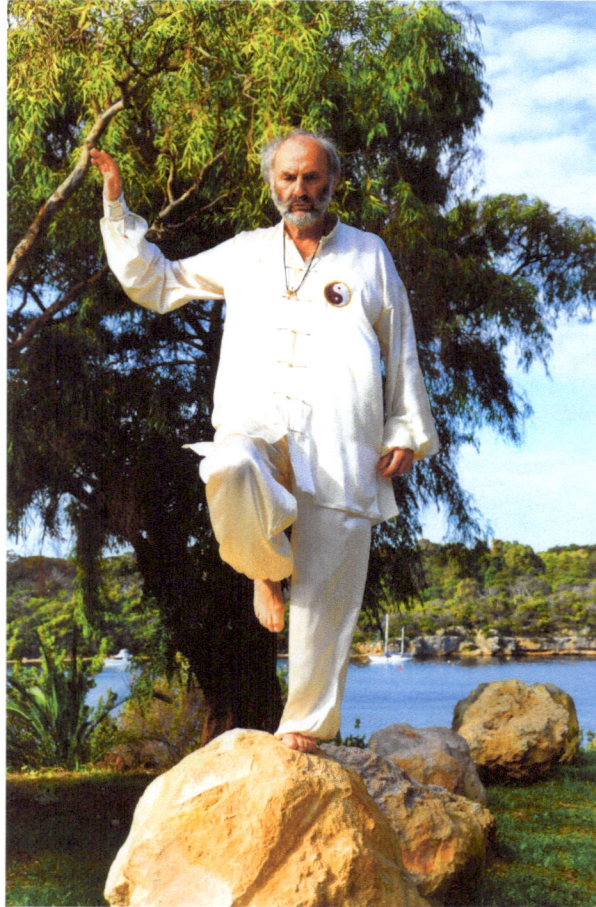

Picture 32. Spleen channel energetic training.
Own work.

Raise your hand and leg at the same time in a movement like a crane's until your hand is level with your temple. Then, slowly lower your arm and leg, keeping both movements in sync. Switch legs and repeat the movement with your right arm and leg. Balancing on one leg can be challenging at first, but it will become easier with practice. Repeat the sequence, alternating between left and right sides several times. The stomach energy channel complements the spleen's energy channel, shown below.

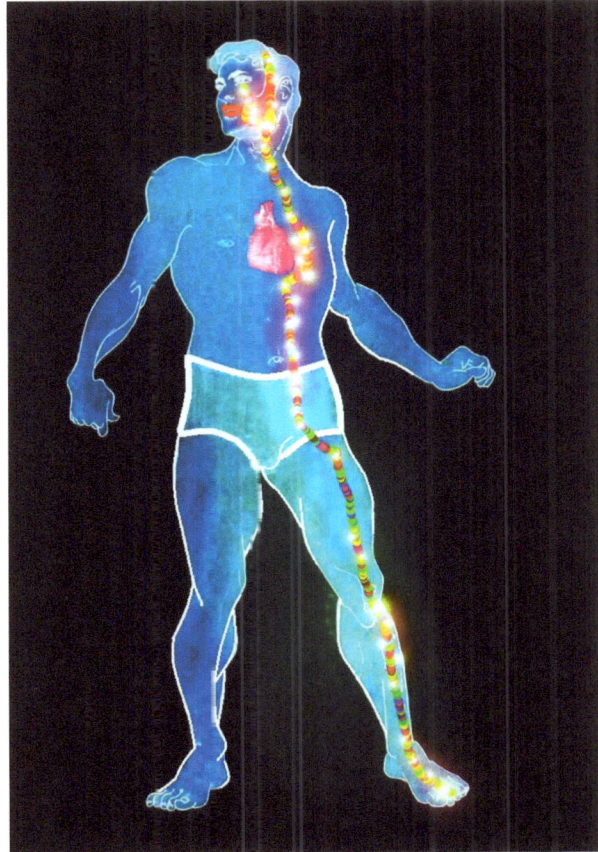

Picture 33. The course of the stomach energy channel.
Own work.

The stomach energy channel builds a functional unit with the spleen energy channel. It starts under the eye and ends between the first and the second toe. It has 45 gateway points.

32

Lungs channel and its energetic training

The lung energy channel originates in the middle of the abdomen at the solar plexus and has two branches. One branch descends to connect with the large intestine, while the other connects to the diaphragm. It then travels upwards into both lungs, continues to the throat, and slants towards the upper chest near the collarbone. From there, it extends to the outside of the body, breaking out below the collarbone, running to the arm and forearm, and ending at the thumb. Along this channel, 11 gateway points are essential for awareness training. Therapists can utilize these entry points for acupuncture or massage treatments.

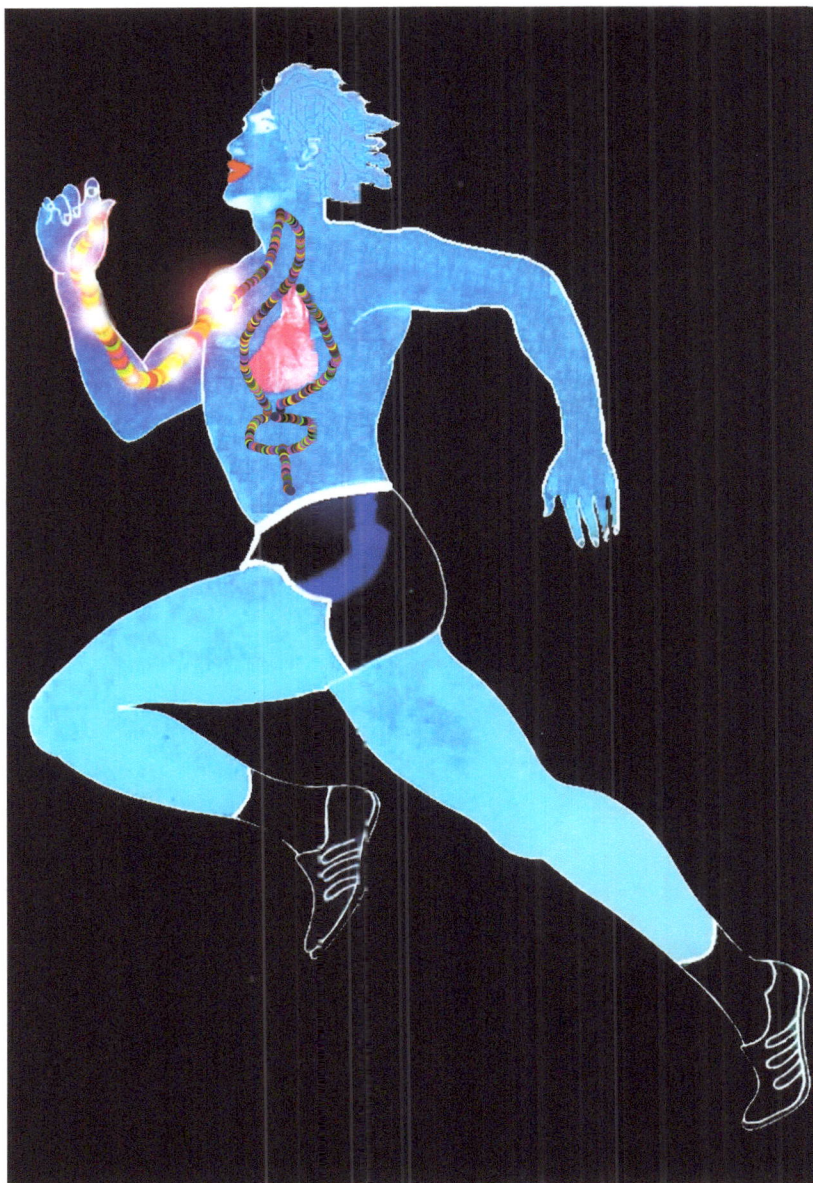

Picture 34. The course of the lunge energy channel.

Own work

Energetic training for the lungs energy channels.

Now, please stand with your left foot towards the direction of the sunset, usually the west, and balance your body weight on the front foot. Spread your arms in a move similar to holding a bow.

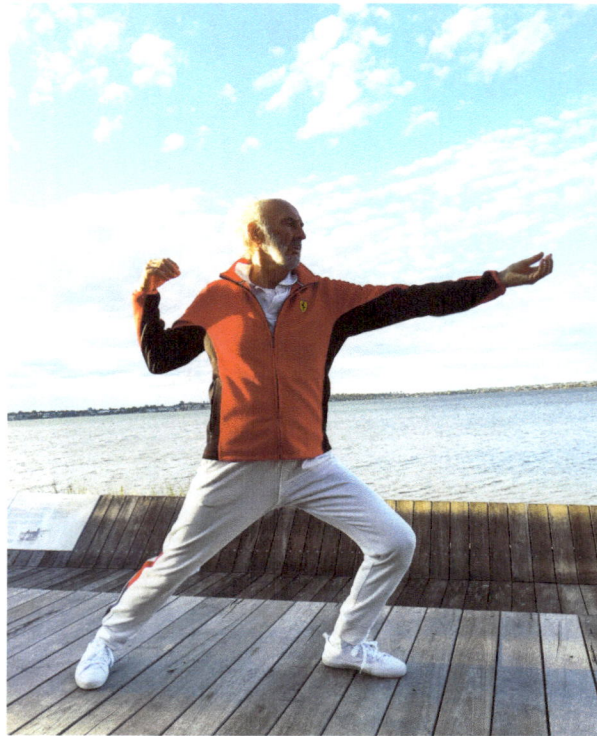

Picture 35. Lungs channel energetic training. Initial position. The left foot is in front of you.
Own work.

Start by assuming the initial position similar to holding a bow, with 80% of your weight on your front legs and 20% on your back legs. Stretch your left arm forward. Next, shift your weight to your back leg and switch the positions of your hands and arms. Rotate your head back so that you end up looking behind you.

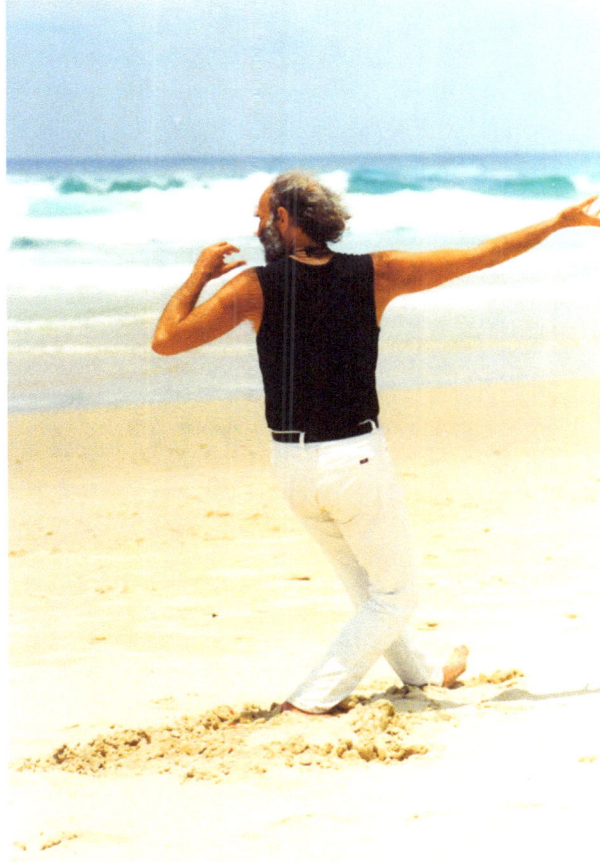

Oicture 36. Energetic training for the lungs channels.
Own work.

Switch your arms at the halfway point of the move. Your hands should meet in front of your face. At the same time, rotate your head, trying to look back, and then return to the initial position. Repeat this sequence several times.

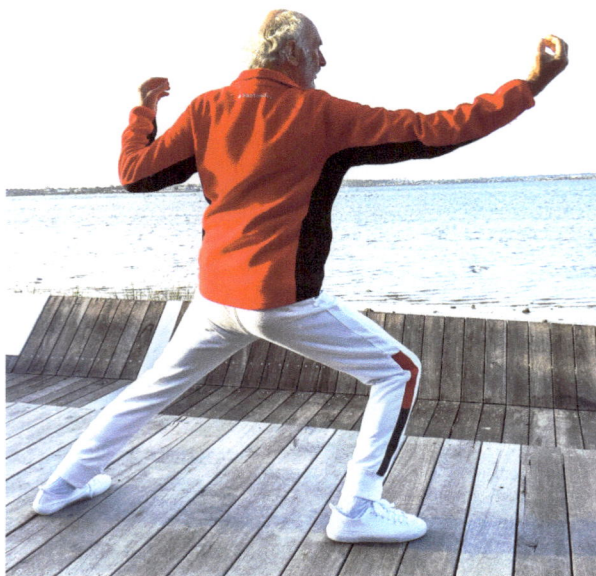

Picture 37. Energetic training for the lungs channels.
Now, it is the right foot in the front of your body.
Own work.

Switch positions with your legs so that your right leg is in front of your left leg. Extend your right arm forward as if holding an invisible bow. Make sure that 80% of your weight is on your right leg and 20% is on your back leg. Then, switch positions with your arms and rotate your head backward, as shown in the picture below.

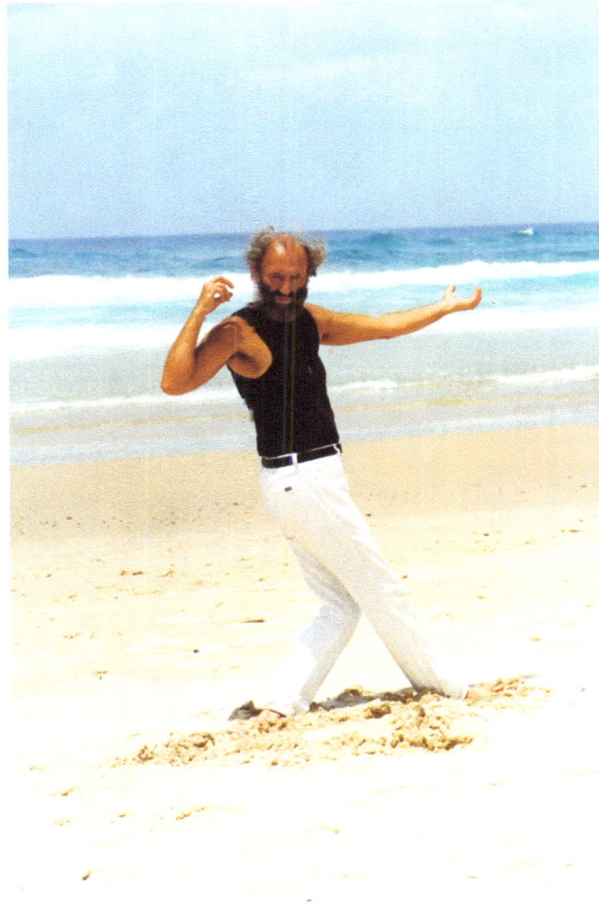

**Picture 38. Energetic training for the lung channels.
Switching the arms.**
Own work.

Your right arm moved back in the opposite direction to the forward-stretched arm, is bent, and the fingers almost touch the upper part of your chest. Perform the movements several times, balancing the body's weight forward and backward.

The large intestine channel supports the lung energy channel. It is displayed below.

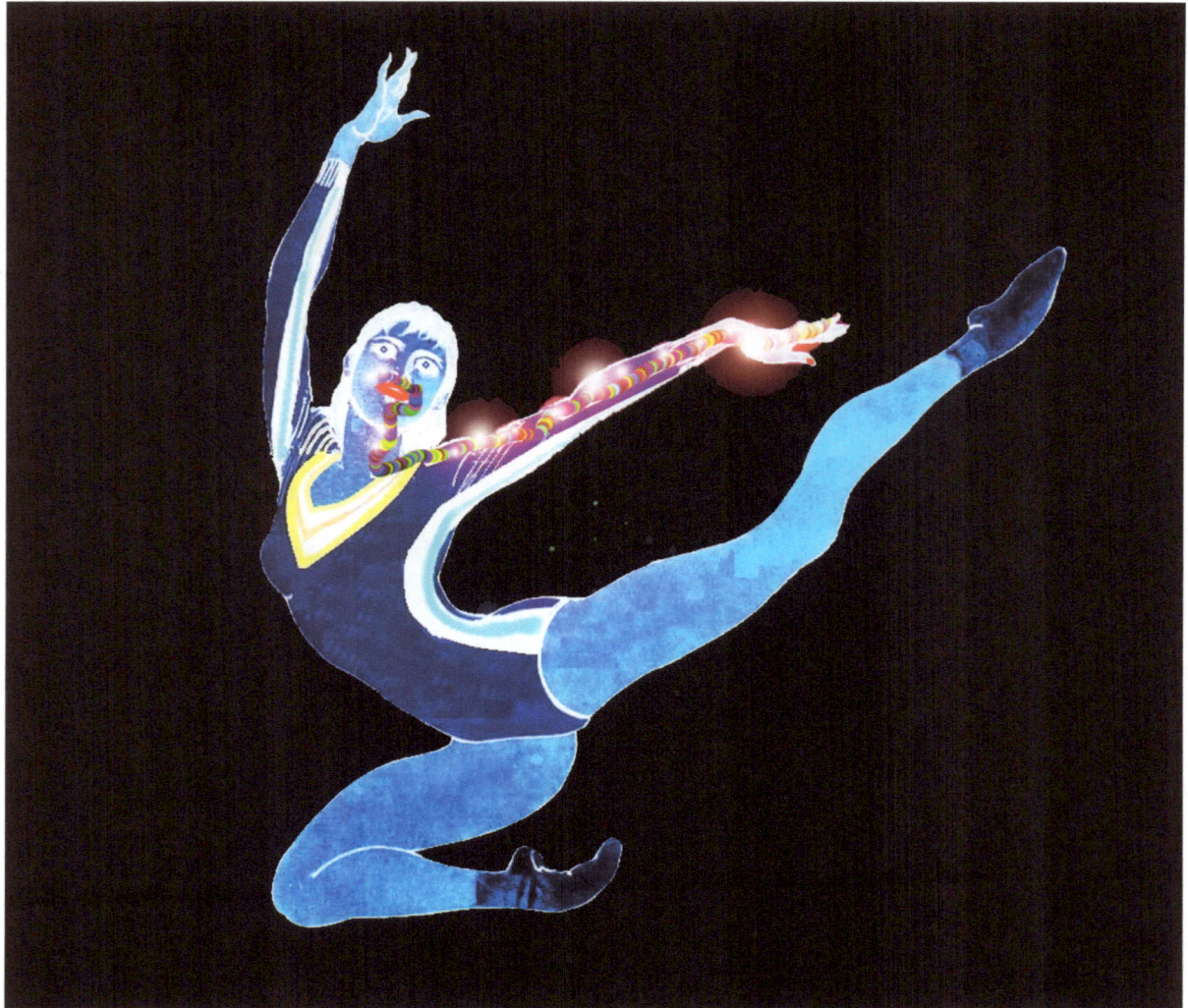

Picture 39. The course of large intestine energy channel.
Own work.

The large intestine energy channel starts from the index finger and ends on oposite side of the face beside the nose. It has 20 gateway points marked with light.

33

Kidneys channel and its energetic training

Kidney energy channel starts in the middle of the forefoot and ends under the collarbone. It has 27 gateway points. It gives internal branches to the end of the spine, the kidneys, reproductive organs, the heart, and the root of the tongue. You can memorize these getaway points for your awareness training. The therapists can use the entry points for treatment with acupuncture or massage.

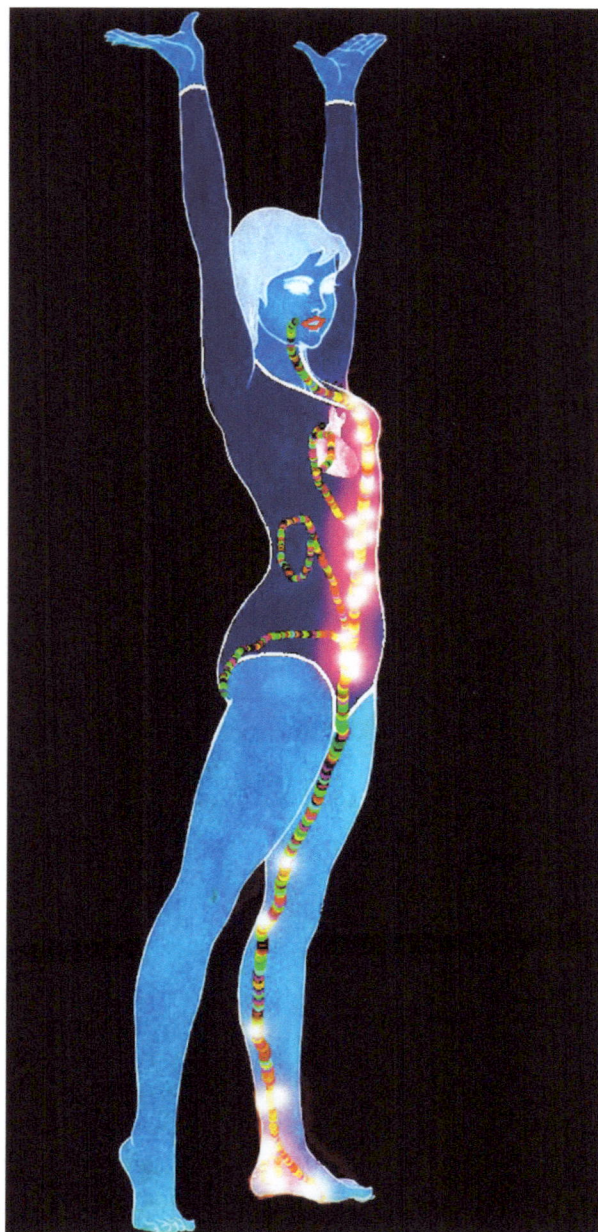

Picture 40. The course of the kidney energy channel.

Energetic training for kidneys channel.

Please take a stand facing away from the sunset direction, typically towards the north.

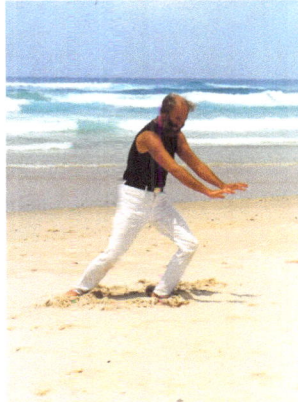

Picture 41. Energetic
trainig for the kidneys
channel,
Own work.

Step forward with your left foot. Keep your body balanced, with about 80% of your weight on your front foot and 20% on your back foot. Move your body and palms towards the ground in a motion resembling the movement of an old mill. Repeat these steps several times.

Then change please your leg and bring the right foot forward. Repeat the moves you just have made with your left leg forward several times.

The urinary bladder channel supports the kidney channel. It is displayed below.

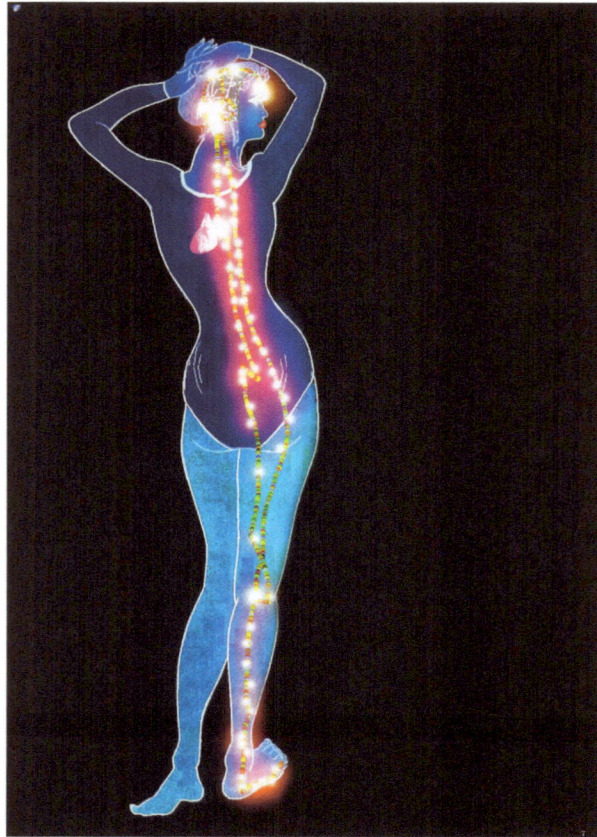

Picture 42. The course of urinary bladder channel.
Own work.

The urinary bladder energy channel starts above the root of the nose, just above the eye and ends at the small toe. It is the longest energy channel in your body. It has 67 gateway points marked in the picture above with light. The therapists can use the entry points for treatment with acupuncture or massage. Own work.

34

Liver channel and its energetic training

The liver energy channel begins between the first and second toes and runs up the front of the body towards the belly. It then loops around the reproductive organs before reaching the liver on the right side of the abdomen. From the liver, the channel branches upward to the heart, the voice box area, mouth, lips, eye, and brain.

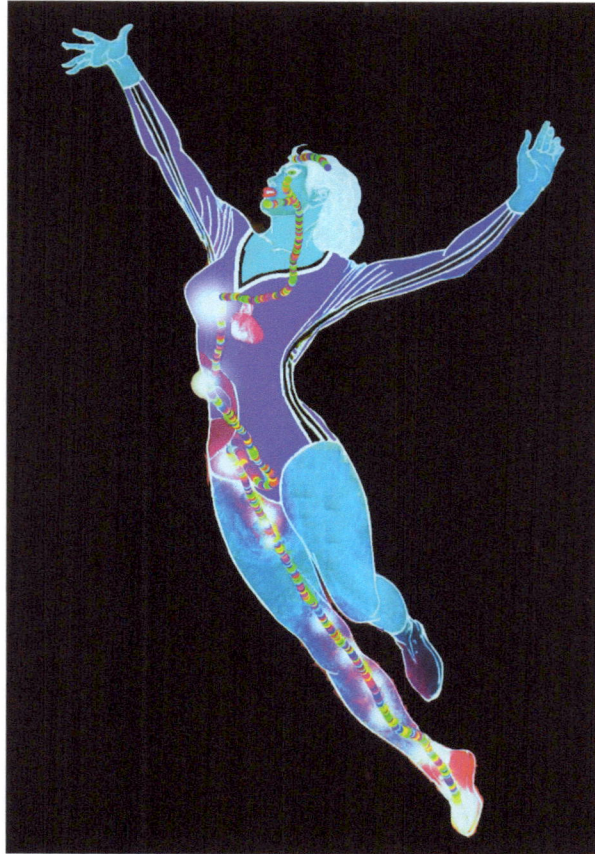

43 Picture. The course of the liver energy channel.
Own work.

The liver energy channel has 14 gateway points that are marked with light. Therapists use these gateway points for interventions such as acupuncture or massage.

Energetic training for the liver energy channel.

Step with your left foot forward, facing the sky where the sun rises, usually the east, and balance the majority of your body's weight on it. Focus on the liver and gall bladder on the right side under the ribcage.

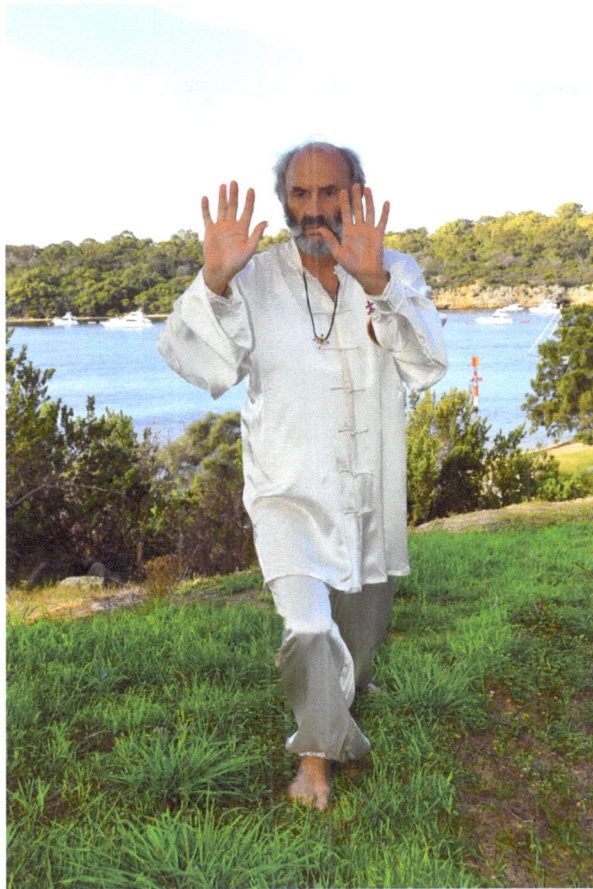

44.. Energetic training for the liver channel.
Own work.

The movement of the hands is like pushing both open hands' palms mentally in front of the body and bringing them back to the point in the direction of the lower belly toward the solar plexus several times. Then, change the position to your right foot in front and repeat this sequence several times.

Remember, it is a mental effort, and the muscles must stay as relaxed as possible. At the same time, balance your body weight forward and then backward.

The gallbladder energy channel supports the liver channel. It is displayed below.

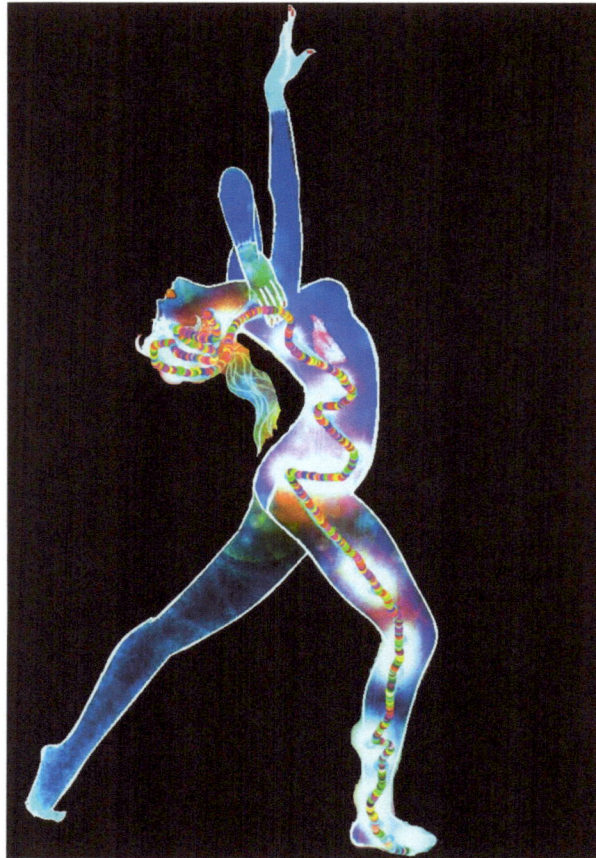

Picture 45. The course of the gall bladder energy channel.
Own work.

The gall bladder energy channel starts at the head close to the eye, about one inch to its outside corner, and ends at the area between your and fourth and fifth toe. It has 44 gateway points marked with light.

35

Acknowledgements

I am immensely grateful for the education and examinations I underwent in traditional Chinese Medicine in Beijing from 1991 to 1997. Throughout that time, I traveled to China frequently with my wife, Angela Rudhart-Dyczynski, and our daughter, Fatima Dyczynski. It's important to note that my wife, Angela, was not just a companion on this journey but the true co-author of this book, and her insights and support shaped its content and direction.

I am thankful for all my acupuncture patients and everyone who has participated in energy channel training with me over the past 35 years. My experiences, ranging from professional to fantastical and occasionally challenging, have made the writing of this book possible.

I want to express my gratitude to Dr. Mary Reinsma, an outstanding and holistic GP, for helping me to stay healthy and fit to write this book.

Furthermore, I am thankful to my Chinese teacher and friends - Dr. Li, who taught me about energy channels and acupuncture; Professor Tianjun Liu, who educated me on Chinese philosophy at Beijing University of Traditional Chinese Medicine; and our translator and interpreter, Sunflower, who is a traditional Chinese medicine doctor.
Traditional Chinese Medicine (TCM) is a well-established and successful concept in traditional medicine. The majority of traditional doctors in China believe in the existence of a channel network known as a system of meridians, which can

be utilized for massage or acupuncture. The fundamental basis of TCM lies in the theory of the five elements and the five internal organs - the heart, lungs, liver, kidneys, and spleen. These organs are vital for the human body as they are the primary source of bio-energy and the ultimate energy generator. TCM takes a holistic approach, with the heart playing a central role as the major organ, governing the entire human body and domesticating the spirit, known as Shen. The meridians and internal organs are believed to be connected to nature and our environment.

One historian of Medicine in China argues that while "meridians" may not be the most suitable term, it has become widely accepted in translations. The term "energy channel" has been adopted in contemporary, traditional medicine, and it seems to better reflect the functionality of the human body.

Dr. Jerzy Dyczynski, MD, MBA, is a medical doctor with a passion for both mainstream and traditional medical approaches. He has been working in the medical field since 1976, specializing in Internal Medicine and Cardiology in hospitals and private practice settings.

In addition to his mainstream medical positions, Dr. Jerzy has over 30 years of experience working as an acupuncturist in public and private healthcare systems in Poland, Germany, Switzerland, and Australia.

In 2008 and 2009, Dr. Jerzy conducted research on Heart-Brain Medicine at Edith Cowan University in Perth and worked as a clinical acupuncturist at the ECU clinic for outpatients.

He earned a Doctor of Medical Sciences and a doctorate in Cardiology in 2002, and has published papers in 70 international journals and delivered over a hundred scientific presentations globally. Dr. Jerzy also completed traditional medicine studies from 1991 to 1997 and received accreditation as an acupuncturist from the University for Traditional Chinese Medicine in Beijing. Dr. Jerzy is also trained in Qi gong traditional gymnastics for health and kung fu martial arts, with over 30 years of experience, and has published two books on the connection between Eastern and Western medicine.

Between 1999 and 2000, Dr. Jerzy attained qualifications in medical quality management for physicians from the Bavarian Medical Council in Munich. His training included moderation, medical leadership, epidemiology, information systems, organizational techniques, quality dimensions, and methods of inter-disciplinary safety models, as well as business process and quality management strategies.

In 2008, Dr. Jerzy graduated from the University of Lueneburg in Germany with a medical MBA in the Management of Outpatient and Integrated Medical Care. Since 2007, he has been living in Perth, Western Australia, practicing as a rural GP and postgraduate researcher in heart-brain medicine at Edith Cowan University.

In 2022, Dr. Jerzy published his book "The Dyczynski Program: Healing the Intelligent Heart," focusing on heart remodeling.